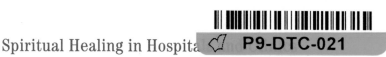
"This book is intriguing and contains true gems—interesting cases, musings, and reminiscences. It is time that our medical system became more open to the data-supported prospect that healing has a clinically valuable effect on patients and seems to trigger effects that the medical system by itself is unable to harness. I am impressed by Sandy Edwards's strength, stamina, and dedication to bring such an ambitious project to fruition."

—HARALD WALACH, clinical psychologist and professor of
research methodology in complementary medicine

"This is an important, deep, and inspiring book. It successfully integrates rigorous evidence-based science with the more subtle approach of spiritual healing. It contains a wealth of heartening anecdotes from patients, clinicians, and spiritual healers. Sandy Edwards is a pioneer in this field having brought spiritual healing directly into an NHS hospital. I warmly recommend her book as required reading for anyone interested in holistic health care and well-being."

—WILLIAM BLOOM, PhD, author of *The Endorphin Effect*

"We are entering an era in which we are rediscovering the ability of conscious intentions to influence distant biological systems. This research is well underway but is little known. Sandy Edwards's research in this field, along with her excellent book *Spiritual Healing in Hospitals and Clinics,* is a major step toward a wider appreciation of this information. The importance of this research extends far beyond healing to the very nature of human consciousness and its origins and destiny. No one can consider themselves an educated citizen in today's world without an awareness of the findings in this important book."

—LARRY DOSSEY, MD, author of *One Mind* and executive editor of
Explore: The Journal of Science and Healing

"Sandy's engaging book tracks how we went from anecdotes to a substantial and rigorous clinical trial that revealed significant findings."

—SUKHDEV SINGH, MD, FRCP, consultant physician

"The results of this research are spectacular. Patients and clinicians should take this work seriously. Sandy Edwards employs both reason and emotion by applying scientific methodology to spiritual healing, challenging a narrow view of biomedicine. The conclusion of her work is clear. Biomedicine must widen its remit to understand, not reject, the mysteries of healing."

—MICHAEL DIXON, LVO, OBE, FRCGP, FRCC, former chair of NHS Alliance, past president of the NHS Clinical Commissioners, and chair of the College of Medicine

"Sandy Edwards first experienced healing when she sought relief from psoriasis. Her book contains the remarkable story of how she went on to set up a healing service in the NHS. It offers a valuable introduction to a complementary therapy that is increasingly being used in the NHS."

—KENNETH DAY, Macmillan clinical nurse specialist

"Sandy brilliantly leads the reader through the scientific evidence confirming that spiritual healing improves health. She skilfully tells her own open and honest story, drawing the reader into how she discovered her own healing hands. I was increasingly eager to read Sandy's diligent research and evidence and had to keep turning the pages to discover the overwhelming benefits that healing can bring to us all and how this story is just the beginning."

—JANET BARETTO, registered nurse, NDND (retired)

"Sandy's book is unique, written in a sympathetic and understanding manner. She takes her reader through a journey of explanation, evidence, and hope and debunks some myths about spiritual healing. By doing so she makes the medical profession sit up and take notice. Having worked with chronic disease management for many years, there can never be too many options for healing available."

—THELMA DEACON, registered nurse

"Sandy's book is very well researched and gives a great insight into spiritual healing. Extensive trials and results are published within the book. A totally different perspective in the treatment of life-changing illnesses."

—JANICE AUSTEN, registered nurse

SPIRITUAL
HEALING
in Hospitals and Clinics

Scientific Evidence that Energy Medicine
Promotes Speedy Recovery and Positive Outcomes

Sandy Edwards

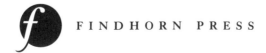

FINDHORN PRESS

Findhorn Press
One Park Street
Rochester, Vermont 05767
www.findhornpress.com

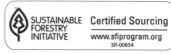

Text stock is SFI certified

Findhorn Press is a division of Inner Traditions International

Disclaimer

The information in this book is given in good faith and is neither intended to diagnose any physical or mental condition nor to serve as a substitute for informed medical advice or care. Please contact your health professional for medical advice and treatment. Neither author nor publisher can be held liable by any person for any loss or damage whatsoever which may arise from the use of this book or any of the information therein.

Cataloging-in-Publication Data for this title is available from the Library of Congress

ISBN 978-1-64411-304-2 (print)
ISBN 978-1-64411-305-9 (ebook)

Printed and bound in the United States by Lake Book Manufacturing, Inc.
The text stock is SFI certified. The Sustainable Forestry Initiative® program promotes sustainable forest management.

10 9 8 7 6 5 4 3 2 1

Edited by Jacqui Lewis
Illustrations by Sandy Edwards
Cover design, text design and layout by Damian Keenan
Cover photos by Marian Vejcik (Dreamstime.com) and Wavebreak Media (Bigstock.com)
This book was typeset in Adobe Garamond Pro, Calluna Sans, and Myriad Pro
with Barlow Condensed and Raleway used as display typefaces

To send correspondence to the author of this book, mail a first-class letter to the author c/o Inner Traditions • Bear & Company, One Park Street, Rochester, VT 05767, and we will forward the communication, or contact the author directly at **www.healinginahospital.uk**

To Roy, Max, and Ben

Contents

"It is believed by experienced doctors that the heat which oozes out of the hand, on being applied to the sick, is highly salutary. It has often appeared while I have been soothing my patients, as if there was a singular property in my hands to pull and draw away from the affected parts, aches and diverse impurities, by laying my hand upon the place and extending my fingers toward it. Thus it is known to some of the learned that health may be implanted in the sick by certain gestures and by contact."

Hippocrates *(460–370 BC), the father of modern medicine*

A Note from the Author

The assertion that spiritual healing is beneficial may seem unbelievable. You may be eager to read the evidence or you may be approaching these pages with acute cynicism. It is healthy to be sceptical but there may be more to gain by being openminded while exploring the possibility.

I hope the evidence and testimonials offered will encourage you to incorporate healing sessions within your normal healthcare regime. Healing is not intended as a substitute for any treatment that has been prescribed by a doctor, and medical help should always be sought for a medical problem.

The information also aims to convey to medical professionals how healing supports conventional care; first and foremost in respect of the benefits to patients, but also regarding cost savings.

You do not need to be ill or distressed to benefit from healing. It can be used to maximize and maintain good health and a positive frame of mind.

By reading this book, I hope you will consider the idea that healing sessions could improve your life. I hope that you will feel inspired to put healing to the test and share your findings with others.

PLEASE NOTE:
The mention of specific organizations, authorities or individuals does not imply that they endorse this book.

Any person whose full name is given in this book is a real person. Either they have given written permission to do so or their statement or story is already in the public domain and the source is referenced.

Any person referred to only by their first name is a real person, but their name has been changed to protect their identity. In some cases, additional details have been changed to add further anonymity.

"The day science begins to study non-physical phenomena, it will make more progress in one decade than in all the previous centuries of its existence."

"My brain is only a receiver; in the Universe there is a core from which we obtain knowledge, strength and inspiration."

"Everyone should consider his body as a priceless gift from one whom he loves above all, a marvellous work of art, of indescribable beauty, and mystery beyond human conception, and so delicate that a word, a breath, a look, nay, a thought may injure it."

"But instinct is something which transcends knowledge. We have, undoubtedly, certain finer fibres that enable us to perceive truths when logical deduction, or any other wilful effort of the brain, is futile."

"So astounding are the facts in this connection, that it would seem as though the Creator himself had electrically designed this planet."

Nikola Tesla (1856–1943)

Foreword

by **Dr Michael Dixon**, LVO, OBE, FRCGP, FRCC

Sandy Edwards' story is one of dogged perseverance on behalf of her patients. Her pioneering work is an example to us all. Having established a hospital healing clinic against all the odds, she then began researching its results, ending with a pragmatic controlled trial of healing, which is about as definitive as it gets. The results of her most recent research are spectacular, though not necessarily surprising for those who have either witnessed or received healing themselves.

It would be as wrong to overestimate the powers of healing as it would be to underestimate them. Some conventional doctors find the whole concept of healing bizarre and scientifically implausible, one example being that of a medical registrar mentioned in the book. Others will dismiss any beneficial effects as placebo. Yet the obvious truth from her research is that healing can provide significant benefit to a substantial number of patients, and she has shown this at a remarkable level of statistical significance.

As stated, the research is pragmatic, and pragmatism would suggest that patients and clinicians should take this work seriously, and especially so if future research also supports its cost-effectiveness.

While Sandy Edwards has taken science just about as far as it can go, her quest is underlaid by deep humanity and compassion. That, after all, is what "healing" is all about. Yet, ironically, this is the very bit that we normally try to exclude in scientific studies when testing the effectiveness of different tablets and procedures.

Central to Sandy's story is the relationship between her and Dr Sukhdev Singh. It reminds me very much of my own relationship with our healer, who first came to my GP clinic well over 20 years ago. My own emotions moved from sceptical fascination to admiration to a deep new learning about patients and my own role as a doctor in healing. Sandy Edwards must be a rather special person to have gained support for healing and for ongoing research in an NHS hospital, against the medical grain and in the way that she did. If my own experience of the work of healers is anything to go by, then I have no doubt that she also healed a number of staff on the way as well.

This is a very impressive book with many important things to tell anyone with open eyes. Some will dismiss the concept of healing and these results on principle. That is not rational. Nor is it rational simply to dismiss everything that cannot be explained. Conversely, Sandy Edwards employs both reason and emotion by applying scientific methodology to a method of healing that is all about feelings and the therapeutic relationship, and which challenges a narrow view of biomedicine.

The conclusion of her work is clear. Biomedicine must widen its remit to understand, not reject, the mysteries of healing with the same open-mindedness shown by staff in the hospital where Sandy Edwards has done her work. This is a story that demonstrates the importance of relationships, empathy, commitment and courage. These are the qualities of a great healer, and Sandy Edwards quite clearly has all these in abundance.

DR MICHAEL DIXON, LVO, OBE, FRCGP, FRCC, is Chair of the College of Medicine (UK), which emphasizes the importance of non-biomedical interventions in health and care, which include social prescription, lifestyle interventions, and complementary and traditional approaches.

Visiting professor at the University of Westminster, London, and at University College London, Dr Dixon is also an Honorary Senior Fellow in Public Policy at the Health Services Management Centre at the University of Birmingham, and an Honorary Senior Fellow Lecturer in Integrated Health at the Peninsula Medical School, Exeter. From 1998 to 2016, he was Chair of the NHS Alliance, now The Health Creation Alliance.

"The most beautiful experience we can have is the mysterious.
It is the fundamental emotion that stands at the cradle of true art
and true science."

"I am convinced that God does not play dice."

"My religion consists of a humble admiration of the illimitable superior
spirit who reveals himself in the slight details we are able to perceive
with our frail and feeble mind."

"Only those who attempt the absurd can achieve the impossible."

$E = mc^2$
E = energy; m = mass; c = speed of light
   [This famous equation says that energy and mass (matter) is
   interchangeable. They are different forms of the same thing.]

Albert Einstein (1879–1955)

1

A Healing Expedition

Spiritual from the Latin "spiritus", means "breath of life"
Healing means "making well"

Healing is a natural phenomenon. After all these years, it continues to amaze me that moving my hands around someone could possibly make a difference to their health and well-being. But there it is. It has been proved to me time and again. The chapters that follow are peppered with patient responses and, despite there being so many, they represent only a fraction of the number of people I have seen. Every other healer will have similar stories to tell and there are many thousands of healers in the UK and around the world, quietly going about their healing work.

If your mind is already teeming with questions about healing, then skip to page 217 for a moment, where you will find all the basics. Any other query is bound to be addressed between here and the back cover. In a tiny nutshell, though, healing is about attuning ourselves to Earth energies and cosmic forces and allowing that unlimited, positive energy to flow through us into the patient. This may sound a preposterous notion, but it seems more than feasible when you examine all of the evidence with an open mind. We might actually be doing this. I do not know. While channelling this energy, and working through the taught sequence of hand positions, we maintain a prayer-like peacefulness that trusts that the work we do will be done for the highest good of all concerned.

There is nothing out of the ordinary about me. If I can learn to give healing then anyone can, if they are sincere and determined. Being more at home with logic and order, I found the world of healing strange but exciting; it opened up a new vista of learning and experiences, leading me to a fresh and wholesome perspective. Discovering healing and developing the skill has been a voyage of awe and wonder that is available to anyone who is prepared to embark.

Every healer I have known talks about sensing energies and seeing colours. They are often surprised to learn that I hardly ever experienced anything extrasensory until after many years of giving healing.

Healing has nothing to do with being psychic or being a medium.

Though I am not interested in developing either of these skills, I do believe that they are valuable gifts when used wisely. But, even if I were a psychic or a medium, the training I received directed against utilizing these senses while giving healing. Our remit is purely and simply to deliver healing. Consequently, when patients eagerly ask if I have picked up any information about them, I invariably have to disappoint. Even if a healer were psychic in any way, it would be against the rules of a reputable healing organization for a healer to glean information about a person without their knowledge. It would be like going through someone's handbag without their permission.

People tend to assume that healers must be particularly kindly and goody-two-shoes types, but this is not necessarily so. However, thanks to the principles that underpin healer training, students become aware of the importance of continually working on themselves, dissolving fears and limitations, forgiving others and transforming the negative thoughts and emotions that lead to stress and worry. Anyone who has taken this challenge to heart will know that it is truly testing and soul-searching stuff. I had a tremendous amount of work to do on myself and I have achieved a great deal, but it remains a lifelong work in progress. Even now, I can be enraged by the diabolical things that people do, and irritated by irksome things that people say. I often quip that I would be a perfect person if nobody upset me! But even that would not be true, of course. Ask anyone I know and they will confirm that I irk as much as anybody else. But rather than dwell upon where people have room for improvement, the point is that character flaws must be no barrier to us becoming effective healers. If we waited until we were perfect or "good enough", nobody would ever learn to give healing.

If there were anything unusual to mention about me, it would be that I was determined to become a healer despite having no sign of a natural ability. So what made me leap into something for which I had no apparent talent?

It was the outcome of my quest to combat psoriasis, a flaky skin condition that was affecting my scalp, causing itching and embarrassment. This had been a constant and tiresome companion since my teens. There is no cure for psoriasis, and steroid cream is the only medical method of gaining temporary relief. Not willing to use steroids, I looked to complementary remedies but achieved no success. Psychology books pointed to deep emotional issues, and I attempted various methods of digging up the offending roots. I felt certain that I was on the right track and made some progress, but it was not enough.

To digress for a moment, hypnosis brought only a small improvement for the psoriasis, but a major breakthrough for smoking. Exactly as the hypnotist said, I have not wanted a puff of a cigarette since that one session. If a hypnotist tells you that you need a course of sessions, find someone else.

During those explorations, I was surprised to be advised by a spiritual healer that I should take up healer training. The act of giving healing, she said, would balance the energies within me that were causing the psoriasis. She recommended the National Federation of Spiritual Healers (NFSH), later to become known as the Healing Trust. I had not heard of the organization before but I felt inspired to follow it up.

For me to resolve to be a healer was like someone who had never seen a cooker deciding to be a chef; plus I expected healing to be in my spare time and entirely unpaid. Also, cooking is within everyone's experience and easily justifiable, whereas healing would be awkward to explain to curious family and friends. Despite the negatives, I felt a thrill at the prospect of training to heal, and I immediately signed up.

I had no sensitivity to the energies that were being talked about on the course, so I found that training to be a healer was like being led down a pitch-black alley without being able to touch the sides. Everyone else seemed to revel in the various sensations that confirmed the validity of what we were being taught. Conversely, I was impervious to such phenomena and just blindly followed instructions. I simply placed my hands in this place or that, precisely as shown, and trusted the process.

My lack of sensitivity seemed to make no difference to the actual effects. Patients gave me as much positive feedback as they did the others. It became evident to me that one could become an effective healer with no natural talent and without needing to sense the energies involved. I supposed that the key to effectiveness must be the amount of passion behind the intent to heal, as I certainly had an abundance of that.

My lack of sensitivity to energies could be due to my being what is termed predominantly "left-brained". When the left hemisphere of the brain is dominant, the person is said to be analytical, objective and logical, which I can identify with. "Right-brained" people, on the other hand, are said to be intuitive, thoughtful and subjective. Neuroscientist Dr Jill Bolte Taylor graphically describes her personal experience of being dominated alternately by the right or the left hemisphere of the brain. As a brain scientist, she was fascinated to witness this while suffering a devastating stroke. Her captivating TED Talk is available to view online.

The softer qualities of right-brained people certainly seem abundant among the countless healers I know. But, again, my being out of step with most other healers made no difference to the positive outcomes for patients.

Incidentally, a few physical phenomena did eventually develop – I describe those later – but it is still a pleasant surprise if I experience anything extrasensory.

Training with the Healing Trust means learning to heal without touching the patient, except for the shoulders and feet. However, we can elect to work with touch, in which case the only additional contact points are the joints of the arms and legs. The patient either sits on a chair or lies on a couch, fully clothed, while the healer encourages them to relax. The session begins with a light touch on the shoulders and then, with hands away from the body, we work downwards, starting around the head and along the trunk of the body. We then work in line with the skeleton, firstly along the spine, then down the arms and legs, finishing with a light touch on the shoulders. The whole process takes about 20 minutes.

For new patients, we explain that they may feel heat, cold, tingling or involuntary muscle jumps, or they might see colours. If they did not know of these possibilities in advance, they might feel alarmed at experiencing something out of the ordinary. Or they might see or feel nothing at all. Everything is normal.

During my training years, a consistent flow of positive feedback from patients compelled me to believe that the training was effective and that healing works. It was astonishing and exciting to find that, simply by my following the method taught, patients reported feeling better. Occasionally, people told me that they had felt physical movements happening deep within the afflicted part of the body, and that it now felt better. More often, people said that their pain had simply disappeared. Others reported that they had experienced a discomfort or an emotion rise up during the session that had then quickly melted away. Tense patients would leave relaxed and those who came in downcast would be uplifted.

I practised my fledgling skills on willing friends and relatives. A colleague at work had been plagued with gout for weeks, and it was getting steadily worse. Walking was excruciatingly painful, but he continued to work full-time. His miserable expression showed that he was unable to find any relief for the agony and that it was getting him down. Although a total sceptic about healing, he was now desperate and prepared to try anything. One Friday lunchtime I gave him a healing session in the office – not the ideal setting in which to unwind, but we had no choice. He was impressed to find that, despite having so much on his mind, he was able to relax deeply. The experience lifted his mood, but the gout remained as painful as ever. I suggested that we try weekly sessions and he agreed.

But on the Monday morning he strode into work all smiles. With amazement all over his face, he described getting out of bed on the Saturday morning and reaching the bedroom door before realizing that his foot was back to normal. And it remained so.

Another surprising healing success concerned my young son. When flying, he invariably had difficulty getting his ears to pop to counteract the changing air pressure. To minimize the pain, we would travel with menthol crystals so that he could sniff the vapour to open his ear canals. Landing was the worst part of the flight, and the prospect of what was to come would spoil any journey for him. During one especially painful descent, I suddenly thought to try healing. There was no time to do the usual whole body circuit, so I simply cupped his ears. The pain disappeared within a minute and, for the first time, he was able to happily watch what was happening outside. He has never had the problem again.

In my very early training days of discovery and wonder, I would eagerly ask each patient what they had felt or experienced during the session and then listen with incredulity to their account. However, I was soon gently corrected and advised that, as a healer, our only remit is to deliver healing. The extent of enquiry afterwards should be limited to "How did that feel?", giving the patient the opportunity to share their experience without feeling pressured.

The range of regular and positive feedback convinced me beyond doubt that healing was making a wonderful difference to people's lives. Further, if I could become an effective healer without the slightest prior ability, and without being able to sense energies, then surely anyone could. Some healing organizations teach that the ability to heal is a natural part of being human – that everyone is a healer, whether they believe it or not. I must have had the capacity all along; it just needed sparking.

After seeing and experiencing how easily people can be helped by healing, I was passionate about letting the world know that it existed. Surely everyone would want to have a slice of this extraordinary pie? But, no. Scepticism stops most people from giving it a chance, and there are many other reasons, too, explained later. A few people decline healing because they think it is against their religion, which I find perplexing.

Healing was illegal in the UK until the early 1950s because, historically, the Christian religion had stamped out and demonized any spiritual practices that bypassed its clergy, which included healing. British law continues to reflect wholesome Christian principles but, partly due to the progress of science, the Church's power has diminished in recent decades, leading to the spiritual liberty that we enjoy today.

Healing was a fundamental part of early Christianity, and remained so for hundreds of years. But when it became an organized religion, many beliefs and practices were modified or rejected. Paradoxically, the resultant Church eschewed healing, even though the most famous healer of all time has to be Jesus. A number of world religions recognize Jesus as an exceptional prophet, which means his teachings must be accepted by all those believers.

Any great leader leads by example and, according to scripture, healing was a major aspect of Jesus' ministry. In addition to his 12 disciples, the Bible says that Jesus empowered 70 others to give healing (Luke 10) and sent them in pairs to at least 41 different destinations. They were to speak with and heal people of all races and creeds. For their work to continue, they must have been empowered to pass this gift on to others, otherwise their mission would have disintegrated when they died.

To send healers to 41 destinations in an area that would have been swarming with traders of all nationalities and faiths, Jesus' intention must surely have been to spread healing across the world, and for it to cascade down through the generations to the present day. Indeed, many cultures throughout history are known to have handed down healing knowledge since ancient times.[1]

Healing can therefore be celebrated as a common link between religions and nations, as well as a spiritual connection between individuals who have a religious faith and those who do not. Healers, and people who come for healing, can be from any religion or none. I know healers who are Catholics or other Christian denominations, Jews, Pagans,

Hindus, Sikhs and Buddhists – and there are bound to be other religious sects represented within the world's healing fraternity.

Even if healers do not belong to a particular faith, they generally do believe in a higher power. But their patients do not need to believe in anything at all. I have seen confirmed sceptics benefit from healing, despite their stonewall attitude. Once again, this highlights the inclusiveness of healing, in that it provides a universal connection between all people regardless of what they believe.

For his television series *The Enemies of Reason*, the well-known debunker and atheist Professor Richard Dawkins interviewed Nicholas Humphrey, Professor of Psychology at the London School of Economics. Humphrey – also an atheist – stated that, even when using traditional medicine, most of the cure is usually from within the patient's own body. He went on to say that, for some patients, alternative medicine can be more effective than traditional treatment and that, therefore, people should not be dissuaded from seeing a healer. The uncut footage reveals further insights, and can be viewed on *YouTube*.

Both the individual giving healing and the one receiving it often experience a glimmer of what some religions refer to as heaven or nirvana. This state of bliss is possible for anyone, religious or not, and brings about "biological homeostasis", the body's natural state of balance and self-repair.[7]

Sometimes, stressed people with no religious faith and with no belief in healing have been astounded to experience a profound sense of elation during their first healing session and have left feeling relaxed, buoyant and invigorated. More normally, people gain confidence with each successive healing session and notice gradual improvements over a series of appointments.

Healer training with a reputable organization is spread over a couple of years to ensure that enough supervision and experience is gained before qualifying. Basic training with the Healing Trust is available to almost anyone, and this initial course provides enough information and practice for attendees to give healing to willing friends. To go any further, membership of the Healing Trust is necessary, and this calls for character references, and also for qualified healers to provide mentorship during the remaining training period. At the end of the programme, patient testimonials and mentor references form part of the final panel assessment.

At the end of my two years, on the way home from qualifying, the idea struck me to apply for a National Lottery grant to set up a voluntary healing centre near my home. Voluntary healing centres are dotted all around the country, but they need to be local enough for people to access them easily. The more the better, I thought, and set about the paperwork. There had never before been a healing centre start-up funded by a grant, so it was a wonderful surprise to open the award letter.

The first healer who agreed to team up knew of an ideal venue for us to use. To avoid the cost of advertising, the town mayor agreed to meet with us and pose for a newspaper article. Our story in the local paper made an impact; it brought 27 patients on our first day, plus a continuing trickle thereafter.

Our team of eight dedicated healers welcomed patients month after month. Volunteers do not grow on trees, and they have a host of other things that they could be doing with their precious time, but these people made our Monday-morning sessions their priority, some travelling quite a distance. Together, we created a friendly and fun atmosphere that our visitors enjoyed being a part of. One new patient stopped mid-stride as he came through the doors, and declared that he could feel the vibes already.

Subsequent grant awards allowed us to produce promotional leaflets, buy exhibition equipment, set up a website, produce an informative DVD, and create a self-help CD called *Sleep Easy & Be Well*.

A hospital in Ohio uses a CD similar to ours, with great success. Cleveland Clinic is consistently ranked as one of the best hospitals in the USA, with patients flying in from all around the world. Some years ago, the clinic implemented a seven-year experiment to see if patients benefited from listening to a guided meditation before, during and after surgery. After just two years, the evidence was so convincing that they halted the trial and put the CD into regular service. Their findings agreed with more than 200 previous studies that guided imagery can help people in the following ways:[3]

- Significant reduction of stress and anxiety before and after surgical and medical procedures.
- Dramatic decrease in pain and less need for pain medication.
- Reduction of side effects and complications resulting from medical procedures.
- Faster recovery and shorter hospital stays.
- Enhanced sleep.
- Strengthening of the immune system and enhanced ability to heal.
- Increase in self-confidence and self-control.

Research shows that patients have been helped by guided imagery when undergoing surgery, chemotherapy, dialysis, in vitro fertilization and various other medical procedures. Given the strength of the evidence over so many years, it would seem obvious to implement this low-cost and effective service throughout any health service. It would be a relatively simple matter to set up and, once installed, the reduced need for medication and ongoing care would more than compensate the investment. More importantly, patients would benefit from a more positive hospital experience.

Many of the beneficial effects listed above have been reported by patients who have used our CD and also by patients who have received in-person healing sessions.

Visitors to our healing group wrote these notes in our comments book:

"Better than fantastic! Wild horses will not keep me away."

"I felt totally rejuvenated, as if I'd slept for a week."

"I am certainly feeling much better after only a few weeks. I can't wait to see what the future holds."

"This has helped me to cope with difficult news. Wonderful healing."

"I always feel low until I get here. After a healing session I feel on top of the world."

"Healing has made me think and feel positively again. I feel relaxed, happy and ready to start taking control of my life again."

"Noticeable differences on a wide range of levels."

"Total peace. What a gift."

"I have felt much better since last week's session. My shoulder has improved and also my eczema. I feel very positive and relaxed and hope that I continue to feel better each week."

"A great experience that is relaxing and energizing. Next day I feel really great. This is the best experience I ever had."

"Wonderful healing. Very relaxing. My mum came recently with a nasty strain, which is completely resolved now due to healing. She is very happy!"

"What a lovely healing. Relaxing and peaceful. Regular healing has helped me to move on with treatment for obsessive compulsive disorder (OCD) and this has become less of a problem for me over the last 12 months. I feel that healing has played a large part in this improvement. I am now 80/20 in control of my life instead of 20/80 before. What a lovely gift, received with thanks."

"The doctor said "no hope" for my painful neck and shoulder and warned that it would get worse. After four healing sessions it has completely healed."

• • •

One of the first patients to arrive at our doors was Chris, who had been off work for three years. He had been unable to take up a new teaching post because of a sudden illness that was followed by a succession of maladies. After a total of 12 healing sessions, this is what he had to say about it:

"When bad health prevented me from taking up a new job, I felt frustrated. A series of illnesses followed, each one seemingly unconnected with the last. It was difficult for my doctor to diagnose as the symptoms kept changing.

"I knew something was wrong but felt that conventional medicine was not an effective response. It was around this time that I saw an advertisement in the local press for spiritual healing. I rang the number and spoke to Sandy, who arranged my first appointment.

"I was unsure as to what to expect. I like to think I have an open mind, but I was concerned that it had something to do with the Spiritualist Church and clairvoyance. I needn't have worried; my first session was very upbeat and uncomplicated. The healers were all very friendly and I found the experience pleasant while not actually being aware of any unusual sensations.

"Sandy explained that one-off recoveries are rare and that the healing process was generally cumulative. It wasn't until three or four sessions later that I could actually feel the healing process taking place.

"After treatment I always felt lighter and more relaxed, tired later in the day and occasionally emotional. I came to realize that healing is not always comfortable; after all, a high temperature is simply a sign of the body healing itself.

"At times, I was aware of specific improvements, while at others I wondered if I was expecting too much. Like watching your hair to see how quickly it is growing, I was only aware of what a difference the healing had made when I looked back after six months of treatment [i e, 12 sessions] and realized that I was, in many ways, a different person. I was physically and mentally stronger, recurrent aches and pains had disappeared, I was sleeping better and, most importantly, feeling optimistic about the future.

"I look upon the healing I have received as a readjustment. I now realize that I was out of balance; I am learning to realign and recover my old sparkle."

After a total of around four hours' treatment, Chris's life was back on track and he was planning to return to work. In comparison to the three years that he had suffered before coming for healing, this was a very small investment of time to achieve such a dramatic change.

• • •

When Chris came to us, our group met only every fortnight. Had we been open every week, as we are now, perhaps he would have been back on his feet in half the time.

If there had been, say, a £6 donation for each of Chris's visits, the total financial outlay would have been £72. This is negligible compared to the cost incurred by the National Health Service (NHS) for his repeated visits to the doctor and for prescriptions over the three-year period. Add to that the expense of sick pay and social security payments for those three years. If the NHS had referred him to our healing centre in the initial stages, or had provided a healer at his doctor's office, it might have been a different story. Chris may well have recovered and returned to work within a few months of becoming ill. With a swift return to work, the national coffers would have made massive savings.

Had Chris not decided to seek healing, he might still be ill now, and perhaps in an even worse condition. The total cost to the taxpayer in healthcare and benefit payments could have been immense. And Chris is only one of many examples.

But healing is about the human story and improving lives. Chris's story highlights the holistic nature of healing in that it helped him physically, mentally and emotionally. The treatments he received from his doctor will have helped some of the symptoms but will not have addressed the cause. Chris enjoyed the healing sessions and positively looked forward to the next one.

• • •

Gwen was another of our earliest patients. By the time she came to us she had been suffering from thyroid problems for five years. Her blood pressure and blood sugar were also problematic and had to be checked every four months. After some regular healing sessions, her thyroid became stable, her blood pressure returned to an acceptable level and her sugar levels improved. She had also been overweight and was delighted to find that she had lost a stone without really trying. She had this to say:

"Healing has helped with back problems, too, which I had a lot of pain with, and had been housebound for 18 months. It is a lot better now. Healing helps me relax and I know that I've benefited in all kinds of ways, not just medically."

Like Chris and Gwen, most people who have experienced healing have done so because they actively looked for it, in the hope that it might help them. But others have had healing "sprung" on them, such as in the following case, where the recipient had no intention of looking for healing and thought it was nonsense.

• • •

Steve had a harrowing accident at work with a circular saw. He cut off the ends of his fingers and they could not be saved. The severed finger ends on his left hand were conspicuously disfigured and excruciatingly painful. Nine months after being discharged from hospital, his situation was no better, and it was around this time that I rang his wife for something.

Steve answered the telephone so I naturally asked how his hand was and, as expected, he gave a glum reply. I knew from his wife how disparaging he was about healing but, nevertheless, I invited him to try a session. Not for a moment did I think that he would accept, but he did. Perhaps I caught him at a particularly weak moment but I grasped the opportunity, and gave him a date and time to come over before he could change his mind. Normally, I would insist that people go to our healing centre but I made an exception for Steve. It was obvious that he would not countenance having healing in public. His wife and I were both agog that he agreed to a session. Hitherto, his wife had been having healing with me in secret because, had he found out, he would have ridiculed her relentlessly.

Steve arrived at our house at the appointed time, nursing his hand and looking at the floor in embarrassment. Shaking his head, he apologized that he did not believe in healing one iota and that it was a mistake that he had come. He said that it was a waste of my time and his. Undeterred by his attitude, I cheerily whisked him through the front door and into our conservatory. There, he dutifully sat on a wooden dining chair, with soft music in the background. Twenty minutes later he felt relaxed, and was bewildered that his hand was entirely pain-free. He admitted that he had enjoyed the session but was mystified. I suggested that he come again the next week and see what else might happen.

● ● ●

When he arrived for his second appointment, his eyes were like saucers as he told me that there had been absolutely no pain in his hand since we last met. He pointed out, though, that there was now a constant tingling in his finger ends, which he found distracting. Could I get rid of it, he enquired. I explained that I do not ask for a particular outcome; I simply give healing and ask that it be for the highest good of all concerned. At the end of the session, Steve was bemused to find that the tingling had indeed disappeared.

At the next session, he told me that the annoying tingling had not returned but that he now had no sensation at all in the ends of his fingers. This meant he did not know what was happening to his fingers unless he looked at them. I conducted the session as normal, again without intending any specific result.

A week later, he was amazed to report that normal feeling had returned and, with wonderment in his eyes, he demonstrated how he could now pick up a pencil with the ends of his truncated fingers. This had been impossible before, due to the pain.

Steve so enjoyed the deep relaxation of a healing session that he continued coming. Over the weeks, he noticed how much more he was enjoying his life, and each week brought news of another beneficial increment. Most surprisingly to both of us, the mushroom-shaped finger ends each became tapered, similar to fingertips, and therefore no longer looked so noticeably different. Also, although they had been rigid and unbending since the accident, all but one finger had now regained full flexibility and grip. One evening, as Steve was leaving our house, he mentally resigned himself to the fact that he would simply have to live with this last finger remaining in its solid state. But before he reached the end of our drive, it suddenly clicked, and has worked perfectly since that moment.

It was only when a colleague of his pointed out how nimbly Steve was handling a tiny nut with his injured hand that he fully realized just how much progress had been made over the course of treatment.

Some while later, he revealed to me that, after the accident, he used to have a morning ritual. Every day he would wake up and immediately remember the horror of the accident. In the vain hope that it was a nightmare, he would look at his hand, and then feel downhearted at the sight of it. He would swear inwardly and a cloud of despondency would hang over him for the rest of the day. Since having the healing sessions, though, he found that he hardly gave the injury a thought.

Steve told me he was so full of vim after each healing session that he felt as though he could cartwheel his way back to the car. He also had the revelation that, without the accident, he would never have discovered healing and gained all the benefits that it had brought. Before the accident his life had seemed a daily drudge, but now he walked with a spring in his step and was laughing more. Although it was an appalling accident, he felt that it had served an important purpose because, as a result, he was now enjoying life. In stark contrast to his previous disparaging attitude towards healing, Steve now confidently recommends healing to anyone, and shrugs off ridicule because he knows that he was once one of those people.

Steve's story reiterates that healing benefits the whole person, not just one aspect. It also shows that people can be helped even if they are totally convinced that healing cannot possibly make a difference. Moreover, his testimony highlights that healing delivered far more than he initially wanted. At the outset, his only concern was to be rid of the incessant pain, but now every aspect of his life was a happier experience than it had been before.

It is rare for me to give someone a series of regular healing sessions and to have a leisurely chat about it with them afterwards. However, I did have the opportunity to do so with Steve, and learned that he had a different experience on every occasion. There was certainly no variation in what I did as I always follow the same routine; and Steve sat in the same place every time. One would presume that the healing energy must be constant. If so, it would seem that any difference could only be caused by either something within him or something within me. My training stressed the importance of healers needing to be in good shape to be a clear channel for healing, and I strive to be so. Whatever the mystery is that causes variance, Steve marvelled at the range of sensations he experienced, and he definitely benefited from every session.

• • •

There was another patient I met enough times to discover just how far-reaching the effects of healing can be. She was a young mother, whom I shall call Liz. Her baby had a distressing complaint for which there was no cure or effective relief. Giving healing at her home enabled us to chat afterwards. It transpired that Liz's father had raised her alone and had been devoted to her, but then circumstances changed and now she had not seen him for several years. After a few healing sessions, Liz found the courage to write a well-crafted letter to her father. We wrote it together, and I delivered it into his hand. But weeks passed and she heard nothing. Perhaps he imagined difficult conversations if they met. Her hopes seemed dashed. But then there was an urgent telephone call to say that he had been rushed into hospital. She raced to his bedside, and anything that had divided them vanished. Thankfully he recovered, and met his son-in-law and grandchildren for the first time. He went on to enjoy being an important part of his daughter's life once more.

Liz's story is another example of the holistic nature of healing. Physically, she and her baby no longer had the medical problems they first came with. Emotionally, her fear of rejection faded enough to allow a positive mental attitude to emerge. She then had the strength to take constructive action and write that letter. Granted, it took a medical emergency for the family to be mended, but sometimes terrible things have to happen for people to realize what is important to them in life.

For me, the unthinkable happened. My sister's first baby, Alice, was diagnosed with a rare congenital condition and given weeks to live. The tragedy shook me to the core. I gave away my business to be able to focus instead on family and on healing. Of course, my anguish was as nothing compared to that of my sister and her husband. Yet despite their unimaginable grief they had the strength and benevolence to think of others. They made arrangements for Alice's corneas to be donated, and these restored the gift of sight to a teenage boy who was rapidly going blind.

Being aware of the depths of suffering to which people can be subject certainly hones the mind. Nevertheless, remaining totally focused for the entirety of a session is difficult for any healer. Only determination and practice develop the level of self-discipline necessary to help make every second of a healing session count. In the delightful words of an Anglican priest I once met, my brain can sometimes feel like a tree full of monkeys. If someone like me can learn to get their unruly jumble of thoughts under control, then anybody can. It remains a challenge for me to keep focused for the entire 20 minutes, but I do my best.

I mentioned earlier my not being sensitive to the subtle energies that other healers speak of but, eventually, I did start experiencing two unusual phenomena. Both are very physical and can be witnessed by anyone.

While giving healing, either or both of my hands might shake now and again, as though some gentle form of electricity is running through them. Confirmation that this is likely to be an effect of healing energy came later when a married couple came to our healing centre.

Relatives normally stay in the reception area, but this man's wife would sit close and watch me give healing to her husband at every appointment. He had never before experienced healing, nor anything like it. Nevertheless, whenever he felt my hands quiver he could clearly see "sheets and sheets of light" behind his closed eyelids. Comparing notes with his wife later, he realized that he could still see the sheets of light when my hands shook, even when my hands were not touching him. I like to think that this involuntary movement in my hands is a sign of particularly strong transformation taking place within the patient, and I therefore continue healing in that spot until the vibrating has ceased.

Very often, I learn later that the patient had a problem in that area, or they might tell me that they experienced an unusual sensation within that part of the body while I was working on them.

The second phenomenon is a clicking sound from my fingernails. When I take my hands away from an area to move on to the next, my fingernails sometimes give an audible "click" that sounds and feels like static electricity. I like to think that these clicks are to do with the electromagnetic field that exists throughout and around each one of us that is fundamental for good health.[4] Every living thing has such a field, including the Earth. Maybe an interaction is occurring between the patient's field and mine. On rare occasions, a multitude of clicks happen all at once, producing a crackle. I take these clicks and crackles as a sign that I should go back to the area that I was working on and resume healing there. When I can move on without hearing a click, I presume that enough healing has been received. Again, people often confirm afterwards that the particular area concerned had been problematic or was the site of an old injury. Since I am not usually aware of subtle energies, these blindingly obvious cues are very helpful!

• • •

As well as organizing the healing centre, I ran a meditation group for those who wanted to learn how to help themselves. Anyone could attend. Some people had neither meditated nor had a healing session before. All the same, people who attended these classes experienced the same range of improvements as those who had one-to-one sessions at our voluntary healing centre.

One woman came along through a chance meeting. She had been sitting on a park bench feeling desolate, missing her husband, who had died a few months earlier. A friend whom she had lost contact with happened to pass by and they struck up conversation. Seeing her so upset, this friend explained about my classes and encouraged her to come along.

After attending for some weeks, this lady wrote:

"Had it not been for meeting an old friend, whom I had not seen for about 25 years, I would not have attended the self-healing meditation group. I had no idea what to expect as I had never heard of this form of therapy. However, I found it very beneficial. I enjoyed the discussions and the meditation was just so very calming. There were lots of tears in the early weeks but the sessions made everything seem brighter. I still have my moments but I am so much more positive now."

I was always on the lookout for ways to introduce healing to more people in need, and a chat with a friend led to my giving a talk to a local motor neurone disease (MND) support group. Our volunteers were subsequently welcomed at their monthly meetings and, despite the disease being harrowing and incurable, a wealth of positive responses flowed. As a result, we eventually became involved with MND's national annual weekend conferences, where members from all over the UK congregated.

Our team of three was constantly busy giving healing to conference delegates, and their feedback was invariably heartening. The following phrases peppered our comments book:

"Wonderfully relaxing."

"Calming."

"Sense of peace."

"Beautiful feeling throughout."

"Feeling of freedom."

"De-stressing."

Others wrote more specific statements, such as:

"I felt heat and energy in areas that were troubled."

"Now breathing properly."

"Headache and shoulder pains gone in five minutes."

"I suffered restless sleep for years until I received a healing session at last year's conference. Since then, I have slept like a log!"

• • •

I was asked to visit a young mother with advanced MND who had reached the stage of being housebound and had only weeks to live. After the first session, her eyes shone while she told me that she no longer feared death and that she now felt at peace about leaving her children without a mother. Until then, she had been utterly distraught.

• • •

Although our work with various self-help groups was enthusiastically received by its members and organizers, one of my main goals was to let the medical world know that healing exists and to have healing made available at NHS venues such as doctors' surgeries and hospitals.

A local hospital hosted the meetings of a thriving support group for breast cancer sufferers. Our volunteer healers were enthusiastically welcomed each month and were kept fully occupied. Feedback confirmed that healing was a great help in many ways to these patients and their families. The organizer of the group ensured that the consultants and medical staff learned of these benefits.

A chance to work directly with medical staff came when another local hospital organized an annual Mind, Body & Soul (MBS) event for the parents of children suffering from cystic fibrosis. There is no cure for this condition, and the affected children themselves were too fragile to attend the MBS event. Instead, the idea was to support their distressed and drained parents. Each year, I joined a team of complementary therapists to help bring attendees ease and comfort. Healing was so popular with both mothers and fathers that my appointment sheet was full every time.

Another opportunity to brush shoulders with the medical world came in 2005. Nursing in Practice organizes national events designed primarily for nurses working in doctors' clinics. I was asked to provide a healing stand at their show at the National Exhibition Centre, a major UK venue. As well as nurses, their delegates included practice managers and other medical staff. This seemed a perfect opportunity for us to introduce healing to healthcare professionals.

When I arrived to set up our stand, I learned that one of the organizers had been suffering from severe back pain for some time. She welcomed the opportunity to try healing and was amazed at the result. The pain disappeared and, throughout the show the following day, she was an enthusiastic ambassador for our stand.

It was the first time that the Nursing in Practice organizers had showcased a complementary therapy, and they were delighted with the interest that we generated. Our team of five volunteers hardly sat down as we delivered taster sessions to over 90 delegates. Almost all of our patients were medical staff, who would now be able to take the message of healing back into their workplace. Hardly any of them had experienced healing before and many were surprised at how deeply they managed to relax. Our comments book was awash with notes of appreciation and descriptions of their positive experiences.

"A most exhilarating experience. Felt wonderful and so relaxed."

"Beautiful colours moving around. Very therapeutic."

"Had a particularly bad night with pain and stress. Much calmer in mind and body now. Ready for the day."

"Wasn't sure at the start but, by the end, felt relaxed and soothed."

"Have not experienced this before but would highly recommend it. Have suffered from a headache all morning. It has gone now."

"I cannot really believe how I felt. It was like a magnet that was pulling [out] my negative energy. I was fully relaxed and will never forget the experience."

"Could feel where the healer was as areas of my body became hot. Felt tired but rejuvenated at the same time."

"Best part of the day! The anxiety I came with has gone."

"Interesting departure from my normal logical thinking. The world is full of mysteries and this made me tingle and relax. Will explore further."

"Wonderful. A real uplifter. Would be great for our patients."

"Thank you so much for giving me so much peace in this busy life of ours. It has been a truly special experience."

"Extremely interesting experience. I would definitely recommend this to my friends and patients."

"Excellent. Felt lovely and the pain in my right foot went away. I would recommend it to anyone."

• • •

These examples demonstrate that the medical professionals had very similar experiences to those related by our other patients. It should be borne in mind that, unlike patients at the healing centre, these people did not come to us actively seeking healing. Most did not realize that spiritual healing existed until they passed our stand. They were not always unwell, yet they noticed improvements.

Many commented that healing might well help support their career by acting as an antidote for the pressures involved in their work. Of course, this would apply to anyone in a demanding job or a stressful situation, whether at home or at work. Being in the medical profession, some of our visitors recognized the potential benefit for their patients and were keen to recommend healing to them.

We exhibited at this show every year for five years, and gave healing to a total of around 500 medical professionals. If they had each introduced healing into their place of work, a doctor's appointment in the region may have been a different experience by now. Stressed staff and sick patients could both have benefited.

Perhaps the answer lies in research findings that nurses are generally open-minded and positive towards healing therapy whereas doctors are most usually not.[5] Offering healing at exhibitions aimed at doctors may help change attitudes and begin to open doors.

A further opportunity to introduce healing to medical staff arose when a city children's hospital hosted conferences for their medical staff to network with complementary therapists.

The theme for their second conference was autism, and presentations had to illustrate how a particular therapy had helped children with this condition. These three children featured in my talk:

My first patient was a four-year-old girl who had no speech and had a habit of pushing people. She seemed to keep herself fully occupied within her own little world. When I entered the living room where she was playing, she gave no indication that I had arrived or that I existed. As with many children, it would have been inappropriate to ask her to sit quietly or lie down while I gave her a healing session in the way that I was taught. Instead, I simply sat on the sofa while she busied herself with toys, and I conducted the healing session in my head, imagining going through the usual routine. Immediately after I had finished, she came over and gave me a kiss. I presumed that this was normal behaviour for the little girl, but her mother's exclamation and expression left no doubt that this was simply unheard of. Kisses were extremely rare, she said, and never given to strangers. We left the child playing and went through to the kitchen for a coffee. While we were chatting, her daughter trotted in with her favourite teddy and gave it to me. Again, her mother was bowled over. A few weeks later, I received news that there had been an uplift in the girl's educational abilities and social interaction. The entire family was happier.

My second subject was a ten-year-old girl who had a nervous, tickly cough that triggered every few minutes. She was on Ritalin and had no eye contact. Although very tense, she was willing to have a healing session in the normal way, sitting on a chair. During that first session, her persistent cough stopped completely, and she left with a permanent smile. A week later, when she arrived for her second session, I learned that she had been smiling all week. Her concentration had improved, the cough hardly existed and she was better all round. In this second session, she saw a bright light in her head that became more comfortable as the session progressed. When she opened her eyes, she said that everything looked a creamy colour initially, then gradually became normal. When she left, she was still smiling. Soon after her two healing sessions, she took her SATs (national examinations in the UK). Although expected to gain Level 3 passes in all subjects, she achieved 4a for maths and 5b for both English and science. These were far above the grades expected by her teachers and family. Her confidence improved so much that she went on to take part in two school productions before starting senior school.

The third child was a delightful junior school lad who was very personable but had difficulty with school work. He was behind in all subjects, especially English, and he was fretting about the approaching SATs. When I arrived at the house, it was a little chaotic. His mother seemed to be late for something, the younger children were squabbling and the parrot was having a fit of squawking. The lad and I were ushered into the front room with the parrot and, to top it all, the boy immediately strode up to the television and switched on his favourite blood and guts movie. Rather than ask him to switch it off, we sat on opposite ends of the settee, him engrossed in carnage and me peacefully conducting healing in my head, the same as with the four-year-old girl. Within a short while, he turned to me and complained that he could not feel anything happening yet. I replied, with a grin, that his attention was probably taken up by the horrors on the screen. Without a further word, he switched the TV off and stretched himself out on the settee in the perfect position to receive healing, eyes closed. I had not made any suggestion for him to do so. Then the whole house became peaceful, including the parrot. It was as though we were the only ones home. Another of the family pets padded in, nestled up against the sofa and fell asleep. Afterwards, the lad announced to his parents that he had enjoyed the session and was happy to have another. When I arrived the next week, his parents told me that he had not worried about the exams since my previous visit. After the second session, he said that he now felt very positive about the SATs, even though they were only a few days away. The following week, he enthusiastically told me how confident he was that his exams had been a success. His parents naturally cautioned him not to be too optimistic, but when his results arrived he was right! His teachers had hoped that he would gain Level 3 for each subject and he did so for English. But he astonished everyone by achieving Level 4 for science and Level 5 for maths. Nobody was more thrilled than he was.

So far as I know, these are the only autistic children that I have given healing to. Considering that the results were so encouraging across all three, healing may be beneficial for other youngsters with this condition. My own very limited experience with children is that, whatever their problem, they noticeably benefit from healing.

My initiatives to bring healing into hospitals and to self-help groups were often welcomed. However, if a key decision-maker was not open-minded about healing, then its introduction would be blocked. Even at places where we were well established, sometimes a new CEO or group leader would arrive and summarily halt our attendance. In all of these instances, they did not listen to patients or offer us an explanation for their decision. It seems unlikely that these situations would occur if it were generally understood that healing is natural and normal. Still greater acceptance could be gained if healing were commonly available in traditional healthcare settings.

Delivering healing at the various hospitals mentioned, and at the Nursing in Practice exhibitions were a step in the right direction towards getting healing noticed by medical personnel, but we needed to bring healing directly into the NHS somehow. We needed a senior person within a hospital or a general practice who was willing to champion our cause. It seemed a tall order, but I kept the thought alive in my mind.

Key Points

- No treatment, whether conventional or complementary, can guarantee a cure, and spiritual healing is no exception.

- Healing helps the whole of a person, not just the problem that is troubling them the most.
- Testimonials from patients and medical professionals confirm the efficacy of healing.
- Babies and children benefit from healing.
- Healing sessions support people who care for others.
- In cases where death is inevitable, healing helps the patient gain peace of mind and acceptance.
- Healing helps relieve emotional issues including bereavement.
- The patient does not need to tell the healer what the problem is.
- A healer who belongs to a reputable organization will not "pick up" information psychically about the patient as this would be unethical.
- Healing can be effective, even when given in a busy and noisy setting, and in a shorter time than usual.
- Healing provides a common, spiritual link between people of diverse races and creeds and those with no religion.
- Anyone can learn to give healing.
- People can learn to self-heal.
- Incorporating healing into conventional healthcare could reduce costs for the NHS, the benefits system and businesses.

2

Healing at the Hospital

One day in 2006, I gave healing to a woman at our voluntary group who had been to us a few times but whom I had not yet met. I was amazed and thrilled when she told me that her hospital consultant had recommended that she come to us. Apparently, he had picked up some of our leaflets from a display stand and had also heard good reports from other doctors about spiritual healing. She said that he had referred a number of his patients to our group and was pleased with the results that he had seen. This was very exciting news. Perhaps he might be open to the idea of making healing available within the hospital.

I wrote to her consultant, Dr Sukhdev Singh, at the Gastroenterology Department of Good Hope Hospital in Birmingham and offered to deliver healing to his patients free of charge. To assure him of the professionalism of the Healing Trust, I detailed the minimum two-year training period, the national standards of training and of accredited tutors, the assessment panels, the professional code of conduct and disciplinary procedures. I also mentioned Healing Trust members who were already well established at other UK hospitals, so he would see that healing was accepted elsewhere.

For example, Ruth Kaye's paid employment as a healer at St James's University Hospital in Leeds (UK) began around 1990, and regular articles in local and national media attest to her ongoing success with patients. As well as giving individual healing sessions on the wards, Ruth runs group sessions at the hospital, where she teaches self-empowerment through meditation and music.[6]

Angie Buxton-King started work as a salaried healer at University College London Hospital (UCLH) in 1999 and, a few years later, was appointed Manager of the Complementary Therapy Team. In addition, Angie and her husband set up a charity in memory of her young son, who had died of cancer. To date, the Sam Buxton Sunflower Healing Trust has financed the first two years' salary of over 25 healers working in cancer departments of hospitals and hospices around the UK. At the end of the two years, the salary commitment has usually been taken over by the recruiting NHS centre.

◆ ◆ ◆

Dr Singh replied to my letter in welcoming terms. He invited me to meet him on the ward where most of his gastroenterology inpatients are cared for. When he stepped forward to shake my hand, my first impression was of his down-to-earth kindliness and I felt that we liked each other from the first moment. In retrospect, he may also have been relieved that I looked and dressed like a hospital administrator and would not look out of place in his clinic. If people imagine that healers wear odd clothes and behave flamboyantly they would most often be wrong.

At that first meeting, Dr Singh introduced me to key members of the nursing and administrative staff on the ward, and we discussed the practicalities of how best to deliver healing to his patients there. An additional suggestion was that I could also give healing to outpatients at his Wednesday-morning clinic.

Now that we had met each other and had agreed upon what was possible, it was up to Dr Singh to gain approval from the hospital's management. Even though it was not a paid position, it took more than 18 months for a decision to be reached by those on high. Perhaps this inordinate delay was because the proposal was so unusual; but, finally, we were able to get started.

To be a volunteer at the hospital, I first had to be interviewed by the coordinator of the Patient Advice Liaison Service. She was fascinated by the concept of healing and curious to know what the patients might experience. I offered to demonstrate on her so that she would have first-hand knowledge of what is involved. Unbeknown to me, her back had been painful for weeks. She was astounded to find that the discomfort disappeared completely within just a few minutes, and it stayed that way. As a result, she became a marvellous exponent of healing and, partly due to her enthusiastic support, we subsequently managed to introduce healers into other departments on the site.

I was surprised to discover that Dr Singh himself led meditation and mindfulness[7] classes for his patients, free of charge and in his own time. It was refreshing and uplifting to meet a medical expert who was proactively including complementary therapies within his provision of care.

• • •

I began work with Dr Singh's patients in August 2007. After their consultation with him, he would suggest that they might benefit from a healing session with me. If they took up the offer, I would lead the person to my room next door.

It is often said that a complementary therapy session helps patients to feel better because they are in nurturing surroundings. However, the room I use at the hospital is a standard, sterile consultation room with no soft music or potted palms. The examination couch in the centre is surrounded by the usual array of medical equipment, and the view through the first-floor window is of the local cemetery.

Another common assertion is that patients feel better only because a complementary therapist takes an interest in them as a person and provides a kindly listening ear. But I exchange just a couple of sentences with a new patient, simply to put them at their ease.

Knowing that the people I see at the hospital have gastric problems, I sometimes lay my hands on their abdomen. When people attend a hospital appointment they anticipate unpleasant invasive treatment so, by comparison, being asked if it is okay to lightly touch inoffensive areas is probably a welcome departure. They invariably agree, and many comment on how comforting it feels.

Working with patients who have been suffering for a very long time, despite best medical care, may seem daunting for a healer. I attempt to maintain a highly positive mindset by means of a variety of methods.

It did not feature in my training, but I believe that the greater a sense of elation and bliss the healer can generate and maintain during the session, the better the outcome for the patient. Whether true or not, it feels brilliant for the healer. Occasionally, I feel intense waves of euphoria and at other times a sudden upwelling of deep emotion that passes through me and goes. When this happens to me, the patient often remarks afterwards that they felt something similar happening to them, and how light and bright they now feel. Others have described having the most amazing experiences, while I was aware of nothing at all. To me, these experiences confirm that powerful healing is occurring.

How can a healer remain optimistic in the face of seemingly insurmountable odds? Physical problems often appear impossible to change. It consequently pleases me to think of ways in which physical improvements may not be as difficult to achieve as we might imagine.

For instance, as easily as cells have moved out of their perfect place for health, why should they not return just as easily? After all, each cell is made up of millions of atoms, and each atom is mostly empty space. The nucleus of an atom is equivalent to the size of a football in the middle of a pitch, with the nearest electron orbiting way outside of the stadium. With such a vast amount of space inside atoms, and with atoms being the building blocks of everything in our world, even the most "solid" piece of rock is, in fact, mostly empty space. So perhaps there really is more room for the cells of our body to manoeuvre than seems possible.

Added to this, astrophysicists know that mysterious elements – dark energy and dark matter – exist that affect the world we can perceive. About 68 per cent of the universe is dark energy and about 27 per cent is dark matter. This means that less than 5 per cent of all that exists is observable. The remaining 95 per cent is only known about because it has an effect on the physical world around us.[8] It does not seem such a great stretch, then, for healers to say that there must be an unknown force called "healing energy" because it has an observable effect on living things.

Scientist James Oschman Ph.D. explains in his book *Energy Medicine* how our cells and tissues respond to energies and vibrations all around us, and discusses the role of natural energy forces within us that work to maintain normal health and well-being.

Scientist Gregg Braden offers a wealth of evidence in his award-winning books to support his contention that there is a field of energy connecting all of creation. He says we communicate with this field through the language of our emotion, and the quality of those emotions reflects in our physical health.

All in all, it seems possible that the physical positioning of atoms, and therefore cells, may be more fluid than we think. Even if it were not actually true, the concept gives me a more limitless mindset when giving healing. But in many cases there seems to be no other explanation.

Probably the best medically documented example is that of Anita Moorjani.[9] Anita had been suffering from cancer for over three years when she was suddenly rushed into hospital one morning, unable to move. Scans showed that the lymphoma had spread throughout her entire body. The oncologist announced that her organs had shut down, and gave her just hours to live. Anita reported later that, while unconscious, she had slipped into a different level of awareness where she experienced great clarity about how life works, as well as an understanding of her own life and its purpose.

She came to understand that "heaven" is a state of mind, not a place, and that her mission was to inspire others with this knowledge.

The next morning, Anita regained normal consciousness. In three days, the tumours in her body, which had been the size of lemons, shrank by 70 per cent. Over the next two weeks, every test came back clear. Her oncologist was baffled. Other doctors who were not involved in her care examined the medical evidence and confirmed that she had returned from certain death. At least one medical expert travelled halfway around the world to investigate, and he reached the same conclusion. Anita's motivational story, which is designed to help others, is related in her book *Dying to Be Me*.

Dannion Brinkley[10] was hit by a bolt of lightning and pronounced dead. On regaining consciousness, he found that he was totally paralyzed and in intense pain. He realized that he was now in the morgue, and thought to be dead. It was only by blowing on the sheet over his face that he was able to alert someone nearby that he was alive. Before this freak accident, Dannion had been a self-centred hellraiser, but during his "death" he had an intense spiritual experience. After he recovered – which took two years, due to appalling burns and impact injuries – he devoted his life to healing and to the care of those approaching death. For more than 20 years he has been actively involved in educating policymakers in the USA on the value of complementary therapies and the need for research. His bestselling book *Saved by the Light* was made into a popular film of the same name.

Denise Linn,[11] when aged 17, was out cycling in the countryside, when an unknown gunman drove past and shot her at close range. A great deal of her abdomen was blown away and she was left for dead on the roadside. It was not thought possible that she could survive such horrific injuries and loss of blood. But while unconscious, she received spiritual revelations, and her wounds subsequently healed at an amazing rate. She has since devoted her life to healing.

Another person who returned to vibrant health despite the odds is Martin Brofman.[12] Martin, who had a high-powered Wall Street career, was diagnosed with a cancerous tumour on his spine and given weeks to live. Surgical removal of the tumour would be so risky that there was hardly any chance of him surviving. With little alternative, he investigated complementary therapies and made a total recovery. As a result of his experience, he became a healer and spiritual teacher.

Donna Eden[13] developed multiple sclerosis (MS) in her teens. MS is a disorder of the central nervous system and, since the nervous system links everything that the body does, it can manifest many different symptoms; it can affect the mind, the body and the emotions, and there is no cure for it. But Donna overcame MS completely by using what she terms "energy medicine". Since then, she has been teaching others how to heal themselves.

Byron Katie[14] experienced a ten-year downward spiral into depression, rage and self-loathing. Normally, it would be unimaginable for someone to recover quickly or completely from the kind of state Byron was in. However, she simply woke up one morning in a state of joy that has remained with her ever since. In this enlightened state of mind, she realized that questioning her stressful thoughts was the key to her recovery. She went on to teach others how to utilize this technique and calls it The Work.

Eckhart Tolle[15] was an intellectual who had spent his life in an almost constant state of anxiety, interspersed with periods of suicidal depression. One morning, when he was 29, he woke up in the early hours with a feeling of absolute dread and the repeating thought that he could not live with himself any longer. When he stopped to think who the "I" was that the "self" could no longer live with, his intellect kicked in and he pondered the problem. By the morning, he was filled with a deep peace and sense of bliss that has remained with him. His bestselling book *The Power of Now* describes his transformation, and guides its readers towards the same realizations.

Norman Cousins[16] was diagnosed with heart disease and told that he had little chance of survival. To take his mind off the constant pain, he watched comedy films. He discovered that ten minutes of genuine belly laughter had an anaesthetic effect that lasted for at least two hours. When the pain-killing effect of the laughter wore off, he would watch more of the film. He believes that laughter cured him and he wrote of his experience in his book *Anatomy of an Illness*, which was later made into a movie. Subsequent research studies have revealed that episodes of laughter help to reduce pain, decrease stress-related hormones and boost the immune system.

Louise Hay[17] was brought up in poverty and had a violent stepfather. She was raped at the age of five and pregnant at fifteen, so it was no wonder that she later changed her name and moved to New York. She eventually found success and happiness, but then was devastated when her husband left her after 14 years of marriage. She turned to religion, where she discovered the transformational power of positive thought and became a popular workshop leader. It was a bitter blow to then be diagnosed with cancer and be told that it was incurable. In response, she declined conventional treatment and began a regime that she believed would rid her body of the disease. Within six months, she was completely healed and lived another 40 years in full health, until she died in her sleep aged 90. She describes her techniques and philosophies in her bestselling book *You Can Heal Your Life*.

Bill Wilson was a successful investment specialist but a drunk. Despite best medical attention, ongoing psychotherapy and a devoted wife, he suffered for decades with this addiction. Eventually, he came to the realization that it was impossible to give up alcohol on his own. While lying in bed, depressed and despairing, he cried out, "I'll do anything! Anything at all! If there be a God, let Him show Himself!" He immediately experienced a bright light, a feeling of ecstasy and a new serenity. He never drank again, and spent the rest of his life helping others to quit drinking. He founded Alcoholics Anonymous, which has helped millions around the world.

* * *

Despite the harrowing situations that these individuals endured, each one of them discovered a key to transformation and went on to lead a healthy and fulfilling life. Further, they had the courage to tell the world their personal stories so that others may be helped and inspired. Although they each use a different method, they all have the same objective.

If just one person can make a physical, mental or emotional recovery, then anyone can. The Institute of Noetic Sciences has compiled a database of thousands of medically reported cases where clinical remission has mysteriously occurred.[18] These recoveries clearly cannot happen outside of the natural laws of physics, chemistry and biology; it must be that we simply do not yet know all of the laws.

Another way that I buoy myself in spite of the apparent odds against a patient's improvement is to trust that the person I am giving healing to is ready to take a quantum leap into wellness and joy. I imagine that they have an internal guidance system that has brought them to this particular place at this precise time so that they can take advantage of this unique healing opportunity. Considering the vastness of space and time, it is easy to envisage that an invisible force could have created this serendipitous "coincidence". Whatever the truth is, generating a positive mindset has to be helpful.

When I first started working at the hospital I also worked with Dr Singh's ward patients, where no session was without interruption. At any time the patient could be visited by a team of doctors, a nurse, the tea lady or visitors. One young man already had a visitor when I arrived, so I told them both that healing was available and offered to come back later if he was interested. He was keen to try it straight away and his mother was agreeable, so she looked on while I worked on her son. Afterwards, he felt that he had benefited from the healing and was more relaxed, and his mother remarked with surprise that her own aches and pains had all disappeared. This is a very common feature of healing.

A very frail woman, who seemed to be a permanent fixture on the ward, told me that she had enjoyed consistently good health until her husband died some years before. She blamed herself for his premature death, even though it was clear that it could not have been her fault. Since that traumatic time, her grief and self-blame had accompanied a downward spiral into ill-health and now she was bed-bound. On the rare occasion like this that I learn the details of someone's background, there is often a story of great loss or anguish that pre-dated the beginning of their illness. Therefore, when giving healing I imagine encompassing the person's invisible past, not just their current physical problems. Medication can be excellent for painful symptoms but it cannot treat a painful past.

Another patient had a similar health pattern, except that her loss was the home she adored. Bereavement can be in many forms.

One colourful pensioner so enjoyed his first healing session at the hospital that he would get a message to me each week to tell me which ward he was now on, and I would go and find him. Upon first sight of me, he would bellow his welcome across the ward and herald "the arrival of the healer". During each session he had strange and wonderful experiences that made his eyes sparkle in the recounting. On my departure, he would call out after me how wonderful he now felt and, thanks to his hearty announcements, a number of patients, staff and visitors came to hear about healing. Sadly, his condition was terminal but healing lifted his spirits no end and he always commented on feeling more physically comfortable.

After several months, I passed this ward work on to other volunteer healers whom I had introduced to the hospital. From then on, I only attended Dr Singh's outpatients clinic.

In my initial months, Dr Singh would make a point of seeing every patient again immediately after their healing session to discover how they had fared. Feedback was consistently positive, which gave him the confidence to progressively reduce the number of patients he called back in.

It must seem extraordinary to a patient, to have their specialist offer them the opportunity of a healing session. Nevertheless, the vast majority took up the offer. Perhaps they did not want to seem rude by turning down Dr Singh's invitation, or maybe they were intrigued. Either way, you will see from my two audits that they most often benefited from just one 20 minute session.

As I had now been a healer for some years, the patient responses seemed perfectly normal to me, but to many of them the experience was astonishing. At the outpatients clinic, it was delightful to see Dr Singh sometimes beckon other consultants over to hear what patients had to say. On one such occasion, he asked the gathered consultants, "How many patients leave our consultations saying, 'That was fantastic!'?" Almost all of the patients I have seen at the hospital were referred to me by Dr Singh. The nursing staff and administrative personnel began actively encouraging patients to see me after they witnessed the difference in some of the individuals.

Very few other consultants at Dr Singh's clinic sent their patients to me. One registrar was initially hesitant but after seeing the difference it made to one of his patients, he referred several more to me. Soon afterwards he took up a promotion at a different hospital and told me that he intended to introduce healing at his new post as soon as he was established enough. At the other end of the spectrum, another registrar never referred a patient to me and told me point blank that medication is the only answer.

Between these two poles, the other consultants were cautiously open-minded, and would send me the occasional patient.

Judging from the few individuals who were referred to me by highly sceptical consultants, a consultant's disbelief did not dampen the patients' positive experience of healing.

• • •

Patients are usually only referred to a specialist when their GP (community doctors in the UK are called general practitioners) has exhausted all of the standard medical remedies for their condition. It follows that Dr Singh's patients would typically have suffered for quite a time before being referred to his clinic. With his specialist knowledge and experience, he naturally has certain expectations of what a patient's prognosis might be and, against this backdrop, he was intrigued that healing seemed to be making a difference. Improvements were often evident immediately after a session and, if patients returned months later for a follow-up appointment, Dr Singh sometimes learned that these positive effects had endured.

• • •

One morning, a young man arrived for his consultation appointment in a hospital wheelchair because he was in too much agony to stand or walk. His wife carried their baby. There was no immediate remedy to alleviate his condition, so Dr Singh suggested a healing session. I wheeled the man into my room where he opted to lie on the couch, but his body was stiffly contorted in an attempt to reduce the pain. Within seconds of my beginning to work, his body began to slowly unwind from its torment, and he melted into a relaxed position, free of pain, and remained so for the rest of the session. He walked out of the unit carrying his baby and left the wheelchair behind.

A year later, he was back for a check-up with Dr Singh. His wife told me that after our healing session a year before, he had been well for four days. However, he had made no attempt to access further healing near to where he lived and turned down the invitation to have another session with me.

There must be a reason why people refuse, or avoid, a chance to improve or get well. I think that the answer is fear, in one guise or another.

One example of this concerned someone I knew whose long-term back pain disappeared after one healing session. Despite the success, she refused a further session some months later when she had another ailment. Eventually, she divulged to me that it had bothered her that healing had solved her back problem, because it challenged her understanding of how the physical world works. If healing is effective, she reasoned, there must be more to life than we can physically see, hear and touch. This prospect seemed like a Pandora's box to her and she was afraid to contemplate the matter further or to have healing again. Years later, though, she did return for additional healing when she was in dire need, and those worries evaporated, along with many others. After that, she was glad to return for healing on a number of occasions. When she was bereaved, she felt that healing supported her immensely. Later on, a whiplash accident left her with recurring shooting pains in her neck and head. She was taking medication and waiting for tests, but the pains disappeared after a few sessions. Then she had a painful growth on her foot that was getting bigger and affecting her gait. After three healing sessions, the lump melted away and she cancelled the operation to remove it.

Another example of someone avoiding healing due to fear was one of Dr Singh's elderly patients. She told me that in her youth, she had seen a healer about a troublesome ailment and had an immediate and full recovery in one session. She was so impressed and overjoyed that she told all her family and friends about it. But they ridiculed her to such an extent that she vowed that she would never go to see a healer again, no matter how ill she was.

It seems strange to me that, despite the fact that her family and friends must have seen the evidence with their own eyes, they refused to acknowledge that healing works.

However, when Dr Singh recommended healing to her, she did agree to a session with me. Constant abdominal pain had made her housebound for some time, but this disappeared during the session and she left the hospital walking normally. The next time I saw her, she told me that, after the previous session, she had caught the bus into town and spent several happy hours shopping, as though she had been let out of prison.

Her escape from pain lasted only for a matter of hours, but it nonetheless demonstrated that the healing had been effective – and a second session gave longer-lasting results – but, again, the pain returned. Unfortunately, logistical issues any further sessions.

A man once initially shied away from having healing because he thought that I might psychically discover secrets about him and his past. I explained to him that no ethical healer would attempt to do so, even if it were possible; it would be prying. Feeling reassured, he accepted healing and felt very much better in mind and body.

Some people refuse healing because their spouse has influenced them against it. Occasionally, I ask patients in the waiting area if they would like a healing session before their appointment with Dr Singh. Female patients often turn to their husband or partner for a decision, rather than make up their own mind. In this situation, the husband almost always dismisses the idea, and his wife then declines the offer. I have not seen this happen the other way about, with a man asking his wife for advice or permission.

It's not only spouses; one woman told her priest how an ongoing, frightening situation in her life had resolved after two healing sessions. Surprisingly, he advised against having healing again and she complied. However, some priests, even in orthodox, conservative churches, do welcome healing.

Additional reasons for refusing healing are more to do with not truly wanting to get well. This category is as much an obstacle for medics as it is for healers. However, healing helps melt away the underlying fears that cause resistance to positive change, and this is another way in which healing can support conventional treatment.

For some, illness brings compassionate care and attention that would otherwise be missing from their lives. Many people appreciate and welcome the kindly interest of medical professionals. Some have little human contact in any other way. Even people with family around them sometimes feel neglected. More than one person has told me that they did not know they were loved by their families until they were diagnosed with a terminal condition.

Others are afraid of the responsibilities that accompany a return to health. While a person is ill, he or she might not be expected to contribute as much as others, whether in the workplace or at home. Some might not be able to work at all, and the longer that someone remains in this demoralizing situation, the more daunting it must be for them to return to the world of work and independent living.

Another reason can be finances. One patient told me that she fell ill and temporarily had to be on sickness benefit; but as soon as she felt capable of work again, she found a job. She felt that a low-paid position would help her rebuild the confidence necessary to return to her previous line of work. However, on pay day, she was shocked to find that her take-home pay was not enough to cover the bills. She was keen to work but could not afford to. Believing that she had no choice, she feigned a relapse of her previous illness and went back on sickness benefit.

Another patient confided that she wanted to be well enough to do what she wanted but at the same time remain disabled enough to continue qualifying for a free mobility car every three years. She had not been able to afford a new car when she worked for a living and did not want to lose this valuable asset.

The onset of deafness provided a secretly welcome benefit for a lady called Verity. When Verity retired, she planned to give up renting her flat near to the office and move in with her sister, Joyce, far away. Neither of them had married and, for financial convenience, they shared ownership of the house that her sister lived in. Verity visited most weekends, but they did not get along at all well. She started to dread the day that she would have to converse with Joyce on an ongoing daily basis. Shortly before retiring, Verity mysteriously lost much of her hearing, thereby giving herself the perfect excuse to minimize communication with Joyce. She was also pleased to find that her sister now had to deal with all the telephone calls and household repairs – chores that Verity was glad to avoid. I gave Verity healing sessions because she enjoyed them, but it was clear that deafness brought too many benefits to hope for a recovery.

Someone else told me that she did not want a healing session because she would feel a fraud if the pain disappeared. She was concerned that people would think that the pain had not been real. Furthermore, she had an imminent appointment with a specialist and did not want to waste his time by arriving with nothing to complain of.

Others refuse healing because they believe that they are not sick enough to warrant it. They feel that others are in greater need and should take their place.

In reality, it is better to tackle a problem while it is small, rather than wait for it to get out of hand. All of us can benefit from healing, even if we appear to the outside world to be happy and healthy. Not one person is physically perfect throughout and totally free of stress and worry in living their lives. Having regular healing sessions is an easy and pleasant method of gaining and maintaining the inner equilibrium that leads to good health.

Some people dismiss the idea of healing because they think it is preposterous, which is entirely understandable. Even after all these years, I sometimes have the same thought myself, sometimes partway through a healing session. How on Earth can placing my hands near to someone's body make a difference to their health or well-being? Yet the feedback from patients continues to corroborate the hundreds of positive comments and reactions that have gone before.

• • •

As well as being a hospital specialist, Dr Singh was also a Senior Lecturer at the University of Birmingham's Medical School. He suggested that I apply to be a tutor for a particular forum where first-year students are introduced to a complementary therapy.

I took up this suggestion, and within a few years of being involved in this forum, I was able to recommend other healers to the organizers. Between us, we introduced healing to around a hundred future medical professionals each year.

Dr Singh also sometimes had medical students in attendance at his Wednesday-morning clinics. Some of these students would watch a healing session in progress and hear what the patient had to say about it afterwards. Others received a healing session themselves and their responses mirrored those of the patients. Hopefully, these future doctors will take this new awareness forward with them into their medical careers.

To help spread the word about healing, I gained a Lottery grant to produce a DVD that explains and demonstrates healing. Dr Singh agreed to be interviewed for it, saying:

I have been a gastroenterology consultant since 1997, seeing patients with abdominal pain, chest pain, anaemia, lack of energy, weight loss, etc. Many of our patients still have symptoms despite our best efforts so, in that situation, I ask patients if they are interested in seeing the healer and, if so, they see the healer following seeing me. We have had this healing service in my clinic for over two years and in that time more than 200 patients have had healing treatment. The responses have been, on the whole, very positive, and for some people very dramatically beneficial.

• • •

Patients also feature on the DVD. Marie Withers, an accountant and business owner, says:

"I was diagnosed with [Stage 4] breast cancer in May 2000. I had a mastectomy in June and I started a radical course of chemotherapy. It was the year end at work and I had an awful lot of things going on and *to be organizing. I set off doing quite well but then, one day, I seemed to hit a wall and I recalled that Sandy was involved in healing and had told me that if I ever needed any help to get in touch with her. One day I got up to go to work and decided I couldn't go. I was a mess. I phoned Sandy and she was available, which was brilliant. I went straight round to her house and began a course of healing, which saved my life, I think.*

"I sat in a chair and had healing that first time, and felt a complete sense of relaxation. I cried but I didn't sob, I didn't move my shoulders and I didn't cry out. My eyes just dripped water for about half an hour, and I felt so good afterwards that I did go to work.

"Physically, the chemotherapy started knocking me about an awful lot. I reacted very badly and spent about two weeks of each month in hospital and Sandy came along to give me healing in hospital, which proved fantastic. It was beneficial, it cheered me up, it made me feel better. I could look more positively at life instead of negatively because, having cancer, everything becomes negative. You question your future. You question your life. Your friends and family find it hard to cope so you find yourself supporting them as much as some of them support you. But when I had the healing I was the one being supported and helped – just me. It was fantastic.

"I still go back to the healing centre. Every now and again, with the pressures of everyday life you get stressed out. You don't give yourself enough time, 'me' time, relaxation time, and when I go to the healing centre it's like an oasis of calm. I can walk in there and start feeling better already. When I've had the healing I feel wonderful."

• • •

Marie mentions how her eyes continually watered during her first session, and I remember us laughing afterwards because her ears were completely full of water! Streaming tears without actually crying is a sign of deep emotional release, and is something that patients often experience.

Over 20 years later, Marie continues to live life in full health and with enthusiasm.

As a result of her own experience, Marie recommended healing to another mother of young children who was having cancer treatment. In addition to the primary tumours, she was worried about some in her neck and shoulders that had newly developed. She was highly sceptical that healing could help, but during that first session, she thought she could feel the lumps in her neck physically shrinking. After that session, the debilitating side effects of the chemotherapy treatment reduced substantially, and within a few visits the lumps in her neck and shoulders disappeared. Ultimately, she made a full recovery.

David Daniels explains on the DVD how he became a healer after receiving healing for an injury.

> *"I had been involved in an accident where I suffered physical injury to my knee joint. I was under pressure at work and quite depressed. I was in quite a bad way, really, and found that healing helped on all those levels at once. It eased my depression and made me feel stronger inside. The pain subsided and it gave me inner strength to cope. I thought that if I could give that to someone else, it would be a fantastic thing to do, and that's why I became a healer."*

• • •

Coral Gardiner had a long-standing medical condition for which she needed regular blood checks at a haematology clinic. She recounts a memorable appointment there:

> *After a blood test, my consultant told me that they had checked my blood a second time because the results had shown it to be normal. I looked at him and thought, "My blood hasn't been normal for 12 years!" The consultant confirmed that my blood was just the same as anyone else's and that they couldn't believe it. I was just through the roof, skipping through the clouds. I could not believe it.*

• • •

Dr John Glaholm, a specialist consultant oncologist, described his own experience of healing on the DVD:

> *I first heard about the [voluntary] healing service [in the Oncology Department] from chemo staff. I have allergy problems myself and one of my colleagues suggested that healing could help.*
>
> *I had a number of sessions lasting 20 to 30 minutes after the end of my clinic, usually very stressful days, that I found tremendously valuable. It provided a tremendous feeling of deep relaxation and well-being that continued. I have found this service particularly*

beneficial and I know that a lot of our patients use this healing service to great effect.

The service is provided by volunteer healers, but it is something that the NHS has to consider taking on board as part of a total package for people with cancer because I think that the benefits are certainly significant. If the healing service were funded by the NHS, it could be expanded so that all of the patients could be cared for this way.

Before having healing I was open-minded about whether it would be of benefit or not. In conventional medicine, we often don't have full answers to problems. You can't just dismiss something because you don't have a scientific understanding of how it might work.

I would certainly recommend it to all patients and would like to see a totally comprehensive service available.

Given the pressures that front-line staff in the health service are under – those who are actively caring for patients in clinics and wards – the stress levels can be extremely high. The psychological burden of dealing with people who are ill is quite considerable and this kind of service would be absolutely invaluable.

Key Points

Members of a reputable healing organization are subject to:

- National standards of training taught by accredited tutors, a minimum training period of two years, final assessment, a professional code of conduct, and disciplinary procedures.
- Healing Trust members do not diagnose, prescribe or manipulate.
- Healing is non-invasive and suitable for all patients no matter how immobile or fragile.
- Unconscious patients can be given healing.
- Pregnant mothers and babies can be given healing.
- There is no limit as to when and where healing can be administered.
- Spiritual healing complements conventional treatment.
- Healing helps dissolve underlying fears that often accompany and/or maintain illness, thereby supporting conventional treatment.

- Healing sessions can be incorporated into any NHS setting.
- Consultants and hospital staff have witnessed the benefit to patients.
- Thousands of medically reported cases exist where clinical remission has occurred that could not be attributed to medical intervention.

3

Effects on Hospital Patients

First Hospital Audit of 75 Patients

Within a few weeks of beginning work at the hospital, I asked Dr Singh if I could conduct an audit of the patients' responses. From the outset, it was clear that people were benefiting from their 20-minute healing session and I wanted to record their comments rather than lose valuable feedback to the ether.

My first set of questions asked how the patient had been over the past week. This included how much pain they had been in, how well they had slept and how good their relationships had been. The second set focused on how the patient felt after seeing the consultant but immediately before the healing session. The third and last section recorded any differences directly after the healing session. A separate sheet of identical questions asked how they were faring one week later.

Although all of the participants would obviously have gastroenterological complaints, I did not want the questionnaire to focus on that particular aspect. Another disorder might be their worst problem.

For instance, I had learned that alcohol and drug addictions can lead to gastrointestinal problems, so some of Dr Singh's patients would be suffering deep emotional problems with far-reaching consequences. Rather than the effect on specific symptoms, I wanted to find out whether healing improved their experience of life. Pain relief, feeling positive, sleeping better and improved relationships seemed the most important elements.

After each question, I gave a scale of one to six so that the participant could indicate the severity of the issue. "1" was clearly labelled as "Excellent" and "6" as "Terrible", but some people were still confused about which end of the scale was which. Some people would start off correctly but then suddenly switch partway down the list of questions. Interestingly, confusion only occurred on the first two sections of the questionnaire – the ones completed before the healing session. Nobody got muddled completing the section that came after the healing session. I suspect that their new clarity of mind was due to being so relaxed.

Healing Questionnaire, Form 1						
To be completed <u>before</u> receiving your healing session	☹ Terrible			Excellent ☺		
Physical comfort over the past week	1	2	3	4	5	6
Relaxation level over the past week	1	2	3	4	5	6
Sleep pattern over the past week	1	2	3	4	5	6
Energy level over the past week	1	2	3	4	5	6
Relationships over the past week	1	2	3	4	5	6
Sense of well-being over the past week (well-being = buoyancy, hope, happiness)	1	2	3	4	5	6
Physical comfort today	1	2	3	4	5	6
Relaxation level today	1	2	3	4	5	6
Energy level today	1	2	3	4	5	6
Sense of well-being today	1	2	3	4	5	6
To be completed <u>after</u> receiving your healing session	☹ Terrible			Excellent ☺		
Physical comfort now	1	2	3	4	5	6
Relaxation level now	1	2	3	4	5	6
Sense of well-being now	1	2	3	4	5	6

Figure 1: Healing Questionnaire 1 – Before and after the Healing Session

Nor did they get mixed up when filling in their "one week later" form in the privacy of their own homes. Again, perhaps this was because they were still feeling calmer and therefore better able to concentrate.

At Dr Singh's request, one of the questions asked patients to give a score for their well-being. The term seemed vague to me, so when I went through the form with patients I verbally explained the meaning before they gave their score for it. When patients completed their "one week later" sheet at home they must have remembered my explanation because their scores were in keeping with the rest of the feedback. This point becomes important later regarding the research results. The questionnaires can be copied and used for official audits or by individuals who wish to plot their own progress.

Healing Questionnaire, Form 2							
To be completed <u>one week</u> after your healing session	☹ Terrible				Excellent ☺		
Physical comfort over the past week	1	2	3	4	5	6
Relaxation level over the past week	1	2	3	4	5	6
Sleep pattern over the past week	1	2	3	4	5	6
Energy level over the past week	1	2	3	4	5	6
Relationships over the past week	1	2	3	4	5	6
Sense of well-being over the past week (well-being = buoyancy, hope, happiness)	1	2	3	4	5	6
A single healing session can be highly effective. However, a series of 6 weekly sessions is often suggested to establish without doubt that improvements have taken place. If such a programme were on offer, would you be interested in participating?							
	Not Likely				Very Likely		
	1	2	3	4	5	6
Any additional comments							

Figure 2: Healing Questionnaire 2 – One Week after the Healing Session

In any event, I ask that the results be forwarded to me (via my website) to enable wider analysis of the expanded data set.

The questionnaire for my first audit was approved by the hospital's Ethics Committee, and I was able to press ahead with my initial survey of seventy-five patients. Figures 1 and 2 present the particular questions posed.

Since conducting the audit, I have improved the scoring sequence by reversing the order and, consequently, the updated questionnaires offered here do not correlate with the bar charts that follow.

Not one of the patients at the hospital was actively looking for healing, so they are in a completely different category from those who come to our healing centre.

People who actively seek healing are willing to make an effort to attend, are prepared to make a donation and are hopeful of a positive outcome. The people at the hospital, on the other hand, probably agreed to have a session only because Dr Singh suggested it to them in positive terms and they did not like to refuse. In addition, it was available immediately, free of charge and in the next room. It could not have been easier for them.

Whilst walking with them for the few steps between Dr Singh's room and mine, I would usually break the ice by asking whether they had ever had healing before. Almost nobody had. Surprisingly, out of these 75 patients, only the tiniest proportion had ever accessed a complementary therapy of any description. In fact, the same ratio applied to all of the patients I saw there. Yet the Department of Health's document *Complementary Medicine Information for Primary Care Groups* paints quite a different picture. It states:

> *In any year it is estimated that 11 per cent of the population visited a complementary therapist for one of ... six named therapies.*

• • •

The "six named therapies" are acupuncture, aromatherapy, chiropractic, homeopathy, hypnotherapy and osteopathy. If healing and popular treatments such as aromatherapy, reflexology and reiki were added to the list, the quoted percentage of 11 per cent would be very much higher. But even the quoted 11 per cent level was in no way reflected among the hundreds of patients I treated at the hospital.

It occurred to me that perhaps people who do embrace complementary therapies are less likely to need a consultant. This might help explain why the national figures are so wildly different from my findings with Dr Singh's patients.

The following series of graphs reflect the scores given by these patients for each particular question. In each of the charts, the height of the columns represents the number of patients. The further the columns are to the left of the graph, the worse those patients felt. The first two sections of the questionnaire were completed directly after the patient had seen Dr Singh. It asked how the patient had been over the past week – the week leading up to their consultation. Black columns in the graphs reflect this information. The second section asked how they felt after their consultation, and grey columns convey the results. Then they had a healing session. The third and final section refers to how patients felt immediately afterwards, and is represented by white columns.

Looking at Figure 3, the black columns illustrate how much pain the patients said they had experienced over the past week. The closer these columns are to the left-hand side of the graph, the more severe their pain was. The column hugging the left-hand side of the graph (position 6) shows that eight people had such terrible pain over the past week that it could not have been worse. Moving to the next black column along (position 5), ten people had terrible pain over the past week but not quite as bad as the people in 6. The next black column is the tallest (position 4), showing that 28 people had very bad pain over the past week but not as bad as the ones in 5. Severity is progressively less as we move towards the right of the graph, until we reach the "Excellent" end. Here we find four people in the last black column (position 1) who said they had been totally free of pain all week.

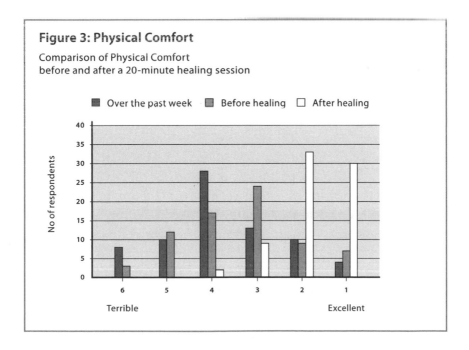

Figure 3: Physical Comfort

Comparison of Physical Comfort
before and after a 20-minute healing session

■ Over the past week ■ Before healing □ After healing

Alongside each black column, the grey ones show how much pain the patient was in straight after their consultation with Dr Singh. They had not yet received a healing session but it is nevertheless clear that the whole set of grey columns has moved towards the right-hand side of the graph, compared to the black ones. This means that the patients were in less pain immediately after seeing the consultant than they had been during the past week. We can see that fewer people are in position 6, where the pain was the worst possible, and a couple more have joined those in position 1, where they had no pain at all. Instead of peaking at position 4, where the highest black column is, the majority of patients in the grey columns are now in position 3, one step closer towards the "Excellent" end. An explanation for this shift is offered in a later section.

Immediately after their healing session, respondents were asked the same question again, and the white columns reveal the difference. Now, nobody is in either of the "Terrible" 6 or 5 positions and only one person is in the 4 column. The two tall white columns dominating the right-hand side of the graph give evidence of a spectacular reduction of physical suffering. We see that 30 people were entirely pain-free by the end of the session (position 1), and a further 33 had hardly any discomfort (position 2). This means that, in addition to the upshift seen after the consultation, a further 47 people jumped into the top two positions, simply from having a 20-minute healing treatment. For some, the pain relief was immediate as well as total. One man had endured incessant pain for over a decade, but almost as soon as I started work, it completely vanished. Understandably, he was overwhelmed with relief. He wept. When pain is relieved, we can expect people to feel better within themselves. The term "sense of well-being" describes how positive a person feels and encompasses such aspects as buoyancy, hope and happiness.

Figure 4 shows that four people in position 6 could not imagine feeling more miserable and despondent than they had been over the past week. Another 15 (position 5) had suffered almost as badly. A further 44 people in columns 4 and 3 had endured respective levels of dejection.

Again, after the consultation with Dr Singh, we see an improvement because the grey columns have nudged towards the right-hand side of the graph, mainly in columns 4 and 3, but especially in 3.

When people were asked the same question after their healing session, it was a different picture. The white columns show that nobody at all was in the extremely gloomy position of 6 and only a few appear in positions 5, 4 and 3. The dramatic leap towards the right of the graph demonstrates a massive uplift for these patients during the healing session. The two tall white columns show that 35 people felt brilliant (position 1), and another 30 felt almost as good (position 2). On top of the gains achieved after their consultation, a further 50 people had moved into the two top positions, simply from spending 20 minutes having a healing session.

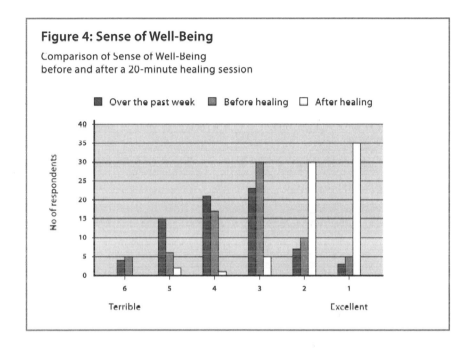

Figure 4: Sense of Well-Being

Comparison of Sense of Well-Being
before and after a 20-minute healing session

Figure 5 measures relaxation, and the black column in position 6 indicates that ten people could not imagine feeling more stressed than over the past week. Another 25 people in position 5 had been almost as bad. At the other end of the scale (position 1), only two people had felt relaxed and calm all week.

Again, after their consultation with Dr Singh, the grey columns slide across the graph towards the right-hand side, signifying an improvement. As before, the white columns reveal how people responded to the healing session. Not one person remained highly stressed and worried (see positions 6 and 5), and only a couple of people appear at the midway points of 4 and 3. Again, the white columns are highly stacked at the right-hand side of the graph. They represent almost every patient; 46 people could not imagine feeling more relaxed, and a further 27 felt almost as good. The majority of the 75 were now in the "could not be better" category instead of only two.

In addition to the gains registered after their consultation, a further 58 people were now in the two top positions, as a direct result of having a healing treatment.

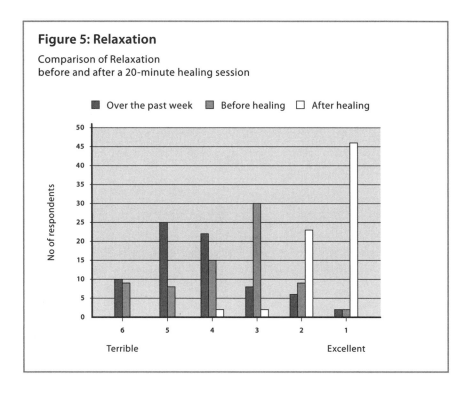

Figure 5: Relaxation

Comparison of Relaxation
before and after a 20-minute healing session

■ Over the past week ■ Before healing □ After healing

When plotting the graphs, I was surprised to find the noticeable shift of the grey columns towards the right-hand side of every graph (Figures 3, 4, and 5). This illustrates the improvements experienced by patients on that particular day in comparison to the whole of the previous week.

The grey columns show how patients were feeling after seeing Dr Singh but before having a healing session. Perhaps patients had been keyed up during the week at the prospect of having to visit the hospital and were now relieved that their consultation was over. Maybe some had not yet met Dr Singh and felt uneasy at the prospect of discussing highly personal matters with someone new. And there might be embarrassing examinations to undergo. Others may have worried about getting to the appointment on time and could now relax. Alternatively, having to focus on getting to the appointment may have diverted their attention from their troubles. Some may have been waiting for test results and, now that they knew the outcome, the stress of uncertainty was gone. Of these, some will have been informed that there was nothing more that the medical world could offer them.

The evident improvements – shown by the grey columns, across all three graphs – could also be due to Dr Singh's natural empathy with patients. Compassion from a doctor is known to elicit a positive effect in the patient and could be due to the Hawthorne effect.[19] The Hawthorne Works in Chicago had commissioned a study to see if their workers would be more productive in higher or lower levels of light. But productivity seemed to temporarily improve no matter what changes were made, and slumped when the study ended. It was concluded that their increased productivity was simply as a result of the interest being shown in them. Likewise, Dr Singh's patients had received no medical intervention during the consultation yet, directly after receiving his attention, reported feeling better than they had been over the previous week.

An interesting point that emerges from the graphs is the obvious link between well-being, relaxation and pain relief; they show that all three aspects improved simultaneously. This phenomenon is made evident to a degree by the grey columns, which register concurrent improvements after the consultation, with all of them shifting a notch towards the "Excellent" end. But after the healing session, it is made entirely obvious by the towering white columns at the right-hand side of every graph.

We all know from personal experience that it is difficult to relax if something is worrying us. When your mind has been put at ease, you physically relax more. It would seem, then, that peace of mind promotes relaxation, and sufficient relaxation brings about pain relief. Scientific evidence to support this idea is presented later.

It could be said that anyone would expect to feel more at peace and relaxed after lying down for 20 minutes. However, of the 75 patients in this audit, 53 chose to add their personal observations and these give a fuller picture of their experience.

The following describe the sensations they encountered during the healing session:

- 10 felt heat or cold.
- 7 felt heaviness or lightness.
- 6 felt tingling.
- 5 saw light of various colours.
- 3 had involuntary muscle movements.

• • •

Patients mentioned these improvements after the healing session while they were completing the questionnaire:

- 21 felt more positive.
- 18 felt relaxed or peaceful.
- 9 stated that pain or discomfort had completely disappeared.
- 6 stated that pain or discomfort had substantially reduced
- 4 stated that pain or discomfort developed during the session but quickly disappeared.

• • •

Although hardly any of my patients knew exactly what to expect, a number of their comments mirrored each other. Regarding the ones that are reproduced below, I have omitted any that simply repeat the observations listed above and have retained those that give some interesting detail. The unabridged list can be viewed on my website.

> *"Wonderful! I feel good for the first time in over 30 years."*
>
> *"I felt warmth in the torso, especially in the stomach and colon. Trembling started in right arm during the session but this stopped when the healer touched that shoulder."*
>
> *"My left side felt empty. Extra healing was given there and I felt complete."*
>
> *"I was aware of lavender light throughout. This has been worthwhile."*
>
> *"A tremor that I have had constantly for a year disappeared now and again during the session. I was aware of heat in the solar plexus*

although the healer's hands were cold."

"I have never sat still and peacefully for so long."

"I did not expect to be comfortable in the chair, due to my back, but it was. I am very impressed."

"I felt warmth during the healing session and can still feel it now. Also tingling in my hands. I felt physical movements in my knees and a tingling. There is no pain in my left knee now."

"I feel that I could sleep for a week! My shoulders feel better now."

"I felt heavy and tingling during the healing session. I felt a pressure on my shoulders, even when the healer took her hands away."

"I am feeling similar to waking up after a long sleep. It felt as though energy was coming in and going out of the base of my feet."

"Involuntary muscle movements set up and also various aches and pains arose but they all disappeared during the session. My eyes watered, too."

"I was most relaxed for what seemed like a long time. It was as though I had been lifted."

"I was aware of coloured circles that gave the impression that something was leaving me, in a positive way."

"I feel ecstatic! I feel like I could run a marathon. I felt tingling throughout my body, which is happening even now. It was especially strong during the session when the healer's hand was on the part of my body that had been problematic."

"Before the session, I was dubious and a little cynical. These feelings have all been washed away now and I feel lighter."

"I had thought that the session would do me no good at all but I definitely feel better."

"Wow, marvellous! This has really helped me. My back pain has disappeared!"

"It was as though a huge lamp was switched on above my head. I felt its heat and saw its light."

One patient was so convinced that I had used heat lamps on her that she insisted on searching all the cupboards!

After concluding the questionnaire, I handed them their "one week later" sheet to complete seven days later. Of the 75 people in this first audit, 32 returned their feedback sheet. In the following series of graphs you will see that the black bars, as before, reflect how this group of patients had felt during the week prior to having healing. Alongside them, the white bars show the difference they noticed over the following week. As before, where the white bars have shifted to the right-hand side of the graph, this indicates improvement.

It was delightful to see in graph form (Figure 6) that so many patients had continued to benefit from reduced pain and less discomfort. Improvement for these people had lasted for at least a week. We had no way of knowing how much longer the benefits remained. They may have been permanent. If there was a weekly pill that was pleasant to take, had no side effects and achieved as much as this, it would surely be popular.

In addition to the improvements shown in these graphs, there will also be people who did benefit but for less than a week.

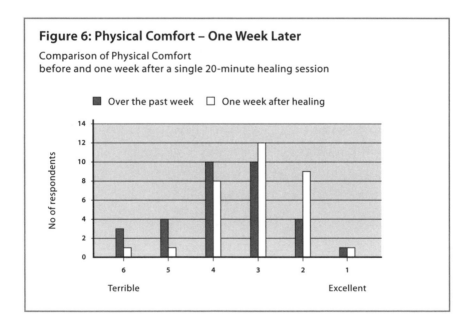

Figure 6: Physical Comfort – One Week Later

Comparison of Physical Comfort
before and one week after a single 20-minute healing session

Figure 7 shows that improvements gained regarding well-being were maintained for at least a week. The black bars in positions 6 and 5 convey the depth of gloominess and bleak outlook experienced by patients during the week before having healing. This state of mind is usually accompanied by a lack of motivation and pessimism. At the other end of the scale, a sense of well-being incorporates peace of mind, buoyancy and hope. Any shift towards the "Excellent" end of the graph conveys an uplift to people's lives.

The evident move of the white bars towards the right-hand side of the graph shows that people continued to feel substantially more upbeat for at least a week after their healing session.

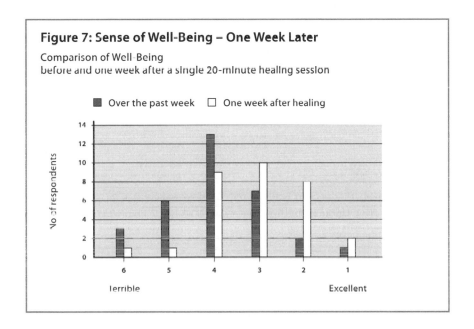

Figure 7: Sense of Well-Being – One Week Later

Comparison of Well-Being before and one week after a single 20-minute healing session

With the black columns in Figure 8 mainly being grouped to the left of the graph, we can appreciate the severity of stress suffered by these patients. A week after the healing session, we see that gains achieved had been maintained. The white columns show that people continued to feel far more relaxed than they had before.

An alarming number of people in our society are on medication to overcome anxiety in its different guises, and many more struggle along without medical support. If healing were made available, it could help to reduce the NHS pharmaceutical bill and bring an improved quality of life to the countless numbers of people who suffer with stress and anxiety.

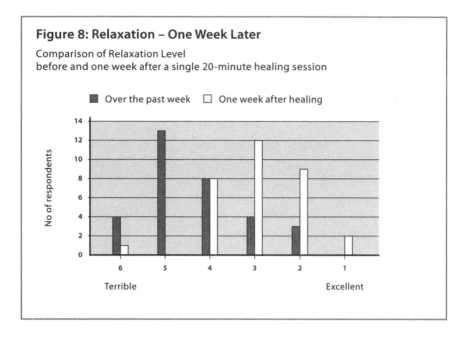

Figure 8: Relaxation – One Week Later

Comparison of Relaxation Level
before and one week after a single 20-minute healing session

It takes a great deal of energy to worry or to be stressed, which must be why we find these states of mind so draining. Stress causes muscle groups to bunch up, most notably in the shoulders or stomach. People often comment after a healing session that they did not realize how tense they had previously been. With so much energy being expended on keeping muscles taut, less energy must be available for day-to-day activities. Also, one would think that tense muscles must restrict the ability of bodily fluids to flow as easily as they should; perhaps this contributes to medical issues.

Figure 9 graphically reveals the marked improvement to people's energy levels one week after their healing session. Again, this benefit may well have lasted longer.

With less anxiety, it should be no surprise that these patients perceived that it was easier to get along with others. Figure 10 displays a noticeable improvement in their personal relationships. Enhanced interaction with family members, friends, neighbours and colleagues is bound to trigger an upward spiral of harmony and vitality.

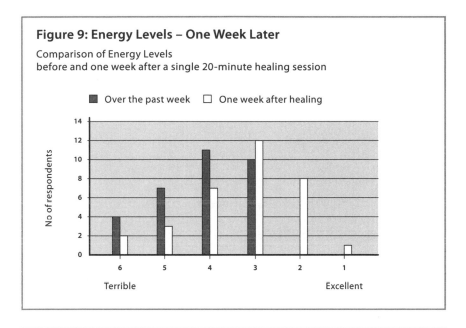

Figure 9: Energy Levels – One Week Later

Comparison of Energy Levels
before and one week after a single 20-minute healing session

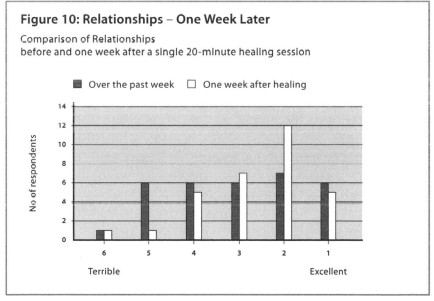

Figure 10: Relationships – One Week Later

Comparison of Relationships
before and one week after a single 20-minute healing session

Figure 11 displays the striking improvement that patients experienced regarding their sleep patterns after just one healing session. The white bars, representing results one week later, have moved considerably towards the right-hand side of the graph, signifying a massive improvement. Again, this uplift may have continued for longer than a week.

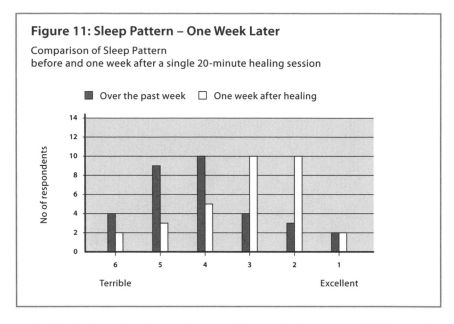

Figure 11: Sleep Pattern – One Week Later

Comparison of Sleep Pattern
before and one week after a single 20-minute healing session

Nobody feels at their best after a restless night but research shows that lack of sleep can be detrimental in a host of ways:[20]

- A study of 56 teenagers over a period of 16 weeks showed that bouts of illness declined when pupils had a longer night's sleep. This reduced school absences, particularly among boys.
- Sleeping poorly may result in a type of brain abnormality that is associated with Alzheimer's disease. Brain images of adults found that those who said they slept poorly had an increased build-up of beta-amyloid plaques, one of the hallmarks of Alzheimer's.
- Regularly getting too little sleep could increase the risk of aggressive breast cancer. Getting six hours or less each night also seems to increase the risk of cancer recurring among post-menopausal breast cancer patients.
- People who regularly sleep for less than six hours a night are 25 per cent more likely to be overweight. Women who sleep less have more abdominal fat, especially those under the age of 50. People who slept less than five hours a night were shown to have belly bulk that often exceeded the medical limit, beyond which coronary diseases become far more likely. Too little sleep affects the production of cortisol and growth

hormones in a way that contributes to increased fat storage in the abdomen.

- Those who sleep less than six hours a night are at greater risk of having a stroke compared with those who sleep seven to eight hours a night. It seems that chronic lack of sleep causes inflammation, elevates blood pressure, raises the heart rate and affects glucose levels, leading to a higher risk of having a stroke.

- Severe sleep deprivation affects the body's immune system in the same way that physical stress does.

- A ten-year study found that sleep deprivation raises average daily blood pressure and increases the heart rate. Through analyzing data from 4,800 people, it was found that those who slept less than six hours a night were twice as likely to have high blood pressure than those getting quality sleep.

- Too little sleep leads to lacklustre and wrinkle-prone skin. Those who had poor quality sleep for at least a month had more fine lines, uneven pigmentation and less elastic skin than good sleepers. Bad sleepers also made slower recovery from sunburn, which suggests that sleep is needed to rectify skin damage. Their skin lost water 30 per cent faster than that of good sleepers, making them more susceptible to wrinkling and environmental damage.

- Quality, unbroken sleep is essential for night-time production of muscle tissue and growth hormones.

- Workers deprived of sleep costs the UK economy an estimated £1.6bn a year, or £280 for each worker.

- Lack of sleep may fuel a junk food habit. It hinders the ability to make healthy choices about food by changing the way our brains function regarding impulse control and decision-making.

• • •

It would seem that some patients sink into a particularly deep state of sleep during a healing session because they exhibit rapid eye movement (REM). During REM sleep, the brain consolidates and processes the information learned during the day and forms neural connections that strengthen memory. It also replenishes the brain's supply of feel-good chemicals like serotonin and dopamine that boost a person's mood during the day. When a person does not get sufficient REM, the brain significantly increases its number of attempts to go into the REM stage while asleep, which suggests that this type of sleep must be crucial.[21]

Not one person whose comments are recorded in this book has mentioned noticing that their eyelids flickered during the session. Although I have seen this occur many times, the patients themselves must be oblivious to it. Behind their closed and flickering eyelids, it is evident that their eyeballs are very active. For some patients these movements occur in short flurries but, occasionally, they can last for the entirety of a session. Whenever I witness someone exhibiting these eye movements during a healing session, they usually report feeling markedly better afterwards. They often mention having had pleasant sensations and sometimes lucid dreams of happy times in their childhood.

According to the Mental Health Foundation (November 2012), more than 30 per cent of the UK population has difficulties with sleep.

Many patients say that they sleep like a log the first night after a healing session. The graph in Figure 11 shows that this welcome effect lasts for at least a week for many people. It may be permanent for some.

• • •

The "one week later" sheet invited additional feedback of any sort and, of the 32 patients who returned their form, the following are some of the comments that go beyond simply saying that they felt better.

> *"I think that my appreciation of my relationships has increased."*

> *"My physical problems did not cease after the session but I felt calmer and more able to cope with them. I would definitely be interested in more healing sessions as I felt so much better after just one."*

> *"I felt relieved in a way. I am hoping that more sessions will make a magnificent change. I am eager to see how I would be after a number of sessions."*

> *"I am very grateful for my extra energy levels. I felt better after one session but would be grateful for more."*

> *"I am really impressed and wish that this was available where I live."*

> *"I had a couple of good days during the week and they were good and relaxed."*

"I have felt calmer about things."

"I slept really well the first night and I feel very positive now."

"Today I find out my results and, considering that this has been on my mind, I have been sleeping well and waking up feeling okay."

"Although my physical condition persists, my feeling of well-being has improved."

"After my healing session, my relationship with my boyfriend was (and still is) good as the healing got rid of my stress and anxiety levels."

"I felt irritable after the session but this lifted the next day and I felt very good."

"I am finding that I can do more things in the day than I could before."

• • •

As well as responses like these that were given on the audit questionnaire, I subsequently discovered feedback from people who had not returned their "one week later" form. For instance:

I bumped into a young man at a Drugs Awareness event. He recognized me and came over to introduce himself as one of the patients I had seen at the hospital. Beaming with confidence, he told me that he had been free of all symptoms since that session and that he was now working. I asked if he had sent in his "one week later" sheet with this splendid news, but he confessed that he had not.

Another of the audit patients had experienced a range of severe problems for over 30 years. After her appointment with Dr Singh, I gave her a healing session. A short while later, she returned for another appointment with Dr Singh. She told me that after that previous healing session, her extreme addiction to coffee had simply disappeared. A hospital letter to her doctor reported "unexplained anaemia resolved", "blood count up" and "stomach and colon normal". All of these improvements confounded the medics.

Another audit patient returned to see Dr Singh for a follow-up appointment and took up the invitation to have a second healing session. With a radiant smile, she confided that, after the previous session several months earlier, she found the courage to learn to read and write. She had been too embarrassed to do anything about it before.

A young woman who had been one of Dr Singh's patients for three years had told me nothing of her condition and was secretly convinced that healing could not make a difference. This is the letter that she subsequently wrote:

> Three years ago I was diagnosed with an autoimmune disease. I began a heavy dose of steroids, along with other forms of medication to bring the illness under control. I had ups and downs and every so often I felt so ill that I would have to stay in bed. But with the loving support of my family I always pulled through, stronger in spirit than before.
>
> Recently, one of my symptoms was what I can only describe as "heavy legs". I was unable to walk with the heavy weight of each leg. I collapsed at work and I was off work for a week. There was no explanation as to why my legs were failing to work properly and blood test results came back normal. I believed that I would just have to grin and bear it. That is, until my consultant suggested that I have a healing session. I have to admit that I was very sceptical as I had never been treated by a healer and had no faith in them.
>
> Sandy Edwards was pleasant, warm and welcoming but I was still wary and decided not to tell her of my ailments or give her any information, just to see the true outcome of the healing session.
>
> I felt what can only be described as lighter. In fact, I went home and took my two crazy dogs for a walk! This was something I had not managed to do for the past two weeks. When I returned home from the walk, my legs were shaky and had returned to the heavy feeling. But the next day my legs began to return to normal. The weight left my legs, and the soreness on the balls of my feet vanished. The following day was as if nothing had been wrong with me and I returned to work.
>
> I did not believe that an alternative method would convert me from a very poorly, non-walking girl to my old healthy self within days. I was sceptical and believed that only a tablet could help me get better but now I am more flexible in my thinking.

• • •

It is important to note that the "one week later" responses and the detailed written accounts, such as the one above, offer more powerful evidence than the questionnaires that I filled in with the patient on the day of the session. People generally like to please and, being face to face with me, some patients may have felt inclined to respond more favourably than they actually experienced. By contrast, the "one week later" information was completed anonymously, in the privacy of their homes, free of external influence, and is therefore more dependable. Statements confessing that their prior disbelief in healing had now been shattered could only be genuine. In addition, the detailed written statements brim with authenticity.

Subsequent to me completing the audits, a young man arrived at Dr Singh's clinic who walked in a strikingly unusual way because one of his legs was lifeless. It had been so since birth, yet he managed to walk without the aid of crutches. He was a complementary therapist and had enthusiastically used natural remedies himself to treat ailments. After his session with me, he was in awe to find that he had been able to feel his leg for the first time in his life. The sensation disappeared when he got up off the couch, but his experience proved that it was possible. It would have been fascinating to see whether further developments might occur but he was unable to attend additional sessions.

No patient I have ever seen, whether at the hospital or anywhere else, has reported a detrimental effect as a result of healing. There were two hospital patients I should mention, though, who seemed gripped with fear at the thought of healing, and whom I therefore did not treat.

The first was a man who had suffered a traumatic event as a child and had been troubled with a range of medical problems ever since. He did not remember anything of the actual incident, even though he had been conscious throughout. Ever since that time, any and every small thing had been causing him acute anxiety. He told me that the thought of completing a form would literally make him faint, so he was not included in my audit. Simply being asked to close his eyes and relax made his head spin. I suggested that he keep his eyes open, but this made no difference.

The second person was a woman who seemed rigid with stress. She told me that she constantly fretted about her family and that she was determined to carry on doing so. Perhaps she felt that worrying was all she could do for her loved ones, because she was physically incapacitated. Personally, I believe that incessant anxiety like this contributes towards physical problems but, whether or not this is true, her family would surely have benefited if she had tried to be a happier person. I attempted to help her relax but, as soon as she closed her eyes, she became extremely dizzy and asked me to stop. It was interesting to note that both of these people suffered extreme dizziness when distressed. Perhaps it is coincidental but I know someone else who loses her sense of balance every time she meets a situation that seems threatening. Although it could be considered, medically speaking, to be vertigo, fear seems to be the underlying cause for all three of these people. As regards the two hospital patients, I sent each of them what is termed "distant healing", which is explained later.

• • •

As a consultant gastroenterologist, Dr Singh has many patients suffering from irritable bowel syndrome (IBS). IBS patients know that their symptoms get worse when they are stressed or worried.

The first scientific evidence that the way we think and feel affects the digestive system was discovered in the 1820s.[22] A young American soldier, Alexis St Martin, was accidentally shot at close range, blasting off the front part of his chest and abdomen. He was not expected to survive such horrific injuries, but a US army surgeon, William Beaumont, fixed what was possible and took the young soldier under his wing. Alexis was tough and recovered but, despite all Beaumont's efforts, a hole remained that led directly into his stomach. A fold like a lid eventually grew over it that could be opened and shut at will. This curious lid made it possible for Beaumont to conduct digestion experiments by putting in different foodstuffs attached to a string that he pulled out at intervals. It was in this way that he discovered that Alexis's digestion was affected whenever the young man was under stress, or worried about something.

If a chemical reaction is known to occur in the stomach due to stress and worry, it seems likely that it is happening throughout the entire body. Different people may have different weak points through which their inner turmoil makes itself manifest. For IBS sufferers, the weak point is clearly their digestive system, whereas others might suffer with something else. Fibromyalgia is a very painful condition that, like IBS, has no physical causes yet flares up with anxiety.[23] Other disorders known to be affected by stress are psoriasis, eczema and hair loss. A traumatic life event or general ongoing stress can trigger diabetes.[24]

Prolonged stress can lead to inflammation; and all medical conditions ending with the suffix "-itis" signify inflammation. Ongoing inflammation can lead to heart disease and cancer.[25] There may be many more illnesses that have not yet been scientifically linked to underlying stress. Low-level but ongoing anxiety probably has subtle effects that overspill in the longer term, like a reservoir that slowly fills until the dam can no longer withstand the pressure.

The Stress Management Society explains the mechanics of stress in detail and offers a range of remedies to try.[26] In a nutshell, anxiety triggers an instinctive reaction known as the "fight or flight" response, which we experience as stress. This "fight or flight" is a survival necessity for when situations truly are dangerous. Hormones are instantly produced to help us to run faster and fight harder, and they also focus our mind solely on the immediate hazard so that we can decide swiftly whether to stand and fight or to run away.

Originally, this reaction was designed for early humans who lived in caves and could have been eaten by wild animals. Few life-threatening events occur in modern-day living, but the same physical reactions continue to occur in response to situations that simply appear to threaten us in some way. Pressure of work, moving house, divorce, children, relationships, traffic jams, unexpected events and financial worries are all contenders. Even a pleasurable event, such as going on holiday, can cause anxiety if the person worries about catching the aeroplane or whether the house might be burgled in their absence.

The more often the "fight or flight" response is stimulated, the more overactive one's hormone production becomes; this can lead to high blood pressure and heart problems. In addition, these hormones make us sensitive, aggressive, excitable, anxious and jumpy. These are all potentially life-saving qualities in an emergency but, in the absence of a real crisis, these attitudes and emotions make life unpleasant. Vigorous exercise can help burn up these energies, but few people are sufficiently active.

Also, when we are focused on our own survival, we view the world as a hostile place and we make decisions for our own good instead of considering others.

Clearly, it is well worth finding ways to combat stress and, as can be seen by the audit responses, healing is experienced as a highly effective antidote. The opposite of the "fight or flight" response is the "rest and digest" state, and patients regularly comment on feeling more relaxed during and after healing. In addition, they often report being more alert and energized, and this makes sense. In light of the above, it seems clear that the massive amount of energy previously expended on feeling stressed had now been freed up for productive and pleasurable activity.

As regards Dr Singh's gastroenterology patients, the "digest" part of the "rest and digest" state of being should be particularly relevant and helpful.

Over the years, I have witnessed a few occasions where a convict has been brought to Dr Singh, handcuffed to prison officers. It is impracticable to offer healing in these circumstances, though I had long wanted to bring healing into prisons. When I mentioned this to Dr Singh, it transpired that he had been giving meditation classes at a local prison on a voluntary basis. He offered to enquire on my behalf about the possibility of introducing healing.

I had in mind the idea of conducting an audit, on similar lines to that of the hospital study, but only with offenders due to be released in six weeks' time. Each one would have weekly healing sessions until their release, and subsequent data would ascertain whether reoffending rates for this group were reduced.

Generally, the public does not approve of criminals being treated to enjoyable activities, but this study could potentially benefit everyone in various ways. Just one incident can cause severe detriment to a victim's life, livelihood and family, so even a minimal improvement in reoffending rates would make a massive difference to the lives of numerous innocent individuals. Add to that the financial burden of prosecuting and jailing the offender as well as the expense of a victim's medical treatment, lost income, sick pay and insurance claims. If six healing sessions helped just one inmate to lead a productive life thereafter, subsequent crimes might be avoided, and the public purse could make some worthwhile savings.

But it took a very long time to get the idea sanctioned and by then, I was no longer able to make the commitment. Perhaps someone will read this and be inspired to take up the idea.

Working with young offenders could be even more rewarding for society in the longer term. They have a longer – and possibly increasingly criminal – life ahead of them. If the attitudes and behaviour of young offenders were to benefit from healing, these young people may go on to raise their own children in a more positive way.

With the intention of helping youngsters, I offered to give ten-minute taster sessions to pupils at a local secondary school during lunchtime. However, it was not practical to give healing as their parents must give prior written permission. Instead, I talked students through a self-relaxation process. I attended each term, once a week, for the next three years on a voluntary basis. The breezeblock room that I was allocated had no windows and seemed the furthest thing imaginable from a haven of tranquillity, but it successfully served its purpose.

A particularly diligent and stressed sixth-former was so impressed by how calm and clear-headed she felt after a session that she wanted the relaxation sessions to be a regular activity for all A-level students. One of the first-year boys seemed beset with silent troubles each time he arrived, and rarely uttered a word. But he would leave walking more upright and with the hint of a smile.

The value of positive relaxation for children has been reported by two schools in Baltimore, USA, since replacing detention with meditation.[27] Many of these young pupils live in deprived areas, and their home life is chaotic and fraught. Since adopting the new strategy, there have been no pupil suspensions, and referrals to the head for disciplinary issues have been rare. The general atmosphere in the schools has improved, creating a better learning environment and increased productivity. Furthermore, students have described how they can now respond in a more positive way to the difficult situations they face at home.

The primary data of my first audit were scrutinized by academics and medical practitioners. No queries were raised, which confirms its integrity. I sent a copy of the audit results to as many people and places as might be interested and there is a copy on my website. The Healing Trust published an article in their national magazine and added it to the research section of their website.

Second Hospital Audit of 192 Patients

I cannot recall what possessed me to begin another audit almost immediately. Perhaps I felt that there was more power in bigger numbers.

My second audit of 192 patients, added to the first, makes a grand total of 267 hospital patients whose responses to healing have been recorded. Hoping to harvest more detailed information from the second audit, I altered the style of the questions, but the feedback was essentially the same. The graphs are almost identical to those of the first audit, so there is little point in reproducing them here. The full details appear on my website. Out of the 192 patients included in this second audit:

- 55 experienced the sensation of heat or cold.
- 52 stated that they now felt more positive.
- 49 people stated that pain or discomfort had disappeared or substantially reduced.
- 30 experienced tingling or rippling sensations.
- 29 experienced involuntary muscle movements.
- 28 experienced seeing light.
- 22 experienced heaviness or lightness.

• • •

Many of the remarks made after the healing session echo those from the first audit, but some add further insights:

"I saw purple light and some dark clouds moved away. Cramps developed but they then disappeared."

"When the healer touched my abdomen, I could feel bloating and a 'letting go' of it. My left wrist and elbow area went very warm. I started coughing during the healing and my eyes were watering."

"I felt benefit immediately. A ripple moved through my body from my pelvis right up through my body."

"I now have total peace of mind. I was very stressed and agitated beforehand."

"I feel 100 times better than I did when I came in. I felt my muscles jump and also tingling. My shoulder went very hot and the pain eased."

"I felt things unknotting."

"The healing made me concentrate on having a positive attitude. I wanted to feel well again."

"Excellent relaxation. This was the first time for me. It gives you a wonderful feeling."

"This was my first healing session. A big weight has lifted and I felt little stars from top to bottom leaving me. I arrived with a cough, which has now settled. The pain in my stomach has gone."

"I felt relaxed, warm and floating. Wonderful! I feel more human. It is like having all your Christmas and birthday presents all in one go."

"The session helped me think about the good in my life."

"Brilliant! Amazing! I have never felt so relaxed in all my life. I feel tingly all over – it is wonderful."

"I have not been so relaxed in months. I had the sensation of a knot in the solar plexus appear during healing that then melted away. Blue and red balls of colour in a grid form appeared in my lower right leg (where an injury had been), which then disappeared. Existing pain in my right side disappeared during the session. I felt very heavy. Emotion surfaced but passed quickly. It was fantastic."

"I felt intense heat across my shoulders and back when the healer's hands were on my abdomen. I felt heat down my left leg, which had been a problem area. It was a very relaxing and positive experience."

"I felt warmth throughout, especially where the healer's hands were in contact. It was particularly hot in my shoulders, abdomen and knees. I had tingles throughout my arms and legs that were different from normal tingles."

"My ankle had been throbbing but that has stopped now and I am not half as aware of my ankle as before. The healer's hands felt as though they were cold – refreshingly cold – but, in reality, the actual temperature of her hands was normal. It was wonderful and revitalizing."

"An ache appeared in my shoulder during the session that then disappeared, accompanied by a sensation of heat. My stomach had bloating and tightness before the session, which significantly released. I was cynical about healing before but now I want to have healing again."

"I have come back for healing as it was so fantastic. For a full five days afterwards, my energy levels were high, I had clarity of thought and I felt peaceful. During this healing session, I felt heat in my tummy and right knee. The tension in my shoulders disappeared."

"I felt as though I was asleep but, at the same time, I was aware that some part of my mind was picking up the words that the healer said. I had been troubled with a burning sensation in my stomach but this disappeared. My right shoulder developed an ache during the session but it then disappeared. I had been sceptical that healing could work."

"I was aware of heat in my neck and head and the discomfort that had been there reduced. I did not want to get off the couch afterwards. I saw lots of blue light. My heart was pounding at the beginning but that has gone now."

"It feels as though a ton weight has been lifted from me. I could not feel the healer's hands on my body. Instead, I was only aware of heat in the areas where there had been pain, which felt like a hot water bottle. I feel great now."

"The problem area felt clogged up before but now it seems more 'spread out' and feels very positive."

"I felt as though I were floating and had a sense of freedom. I felt as though I was running through a field of knee-high flowers."

"I feel energized, positive and relaxed. The healer's hand vibrated when it was on my left shoulder, which I had not told her had been painful recently. I was aware of purple, bubbly clouds around my head."

"Mind-blowing! I felt tingling sensations, as though negativity was being brought out. I feel a bit stronger now."

"I felt as though I had been in a deep sleep although I could hear people and traffic outside. I feel a lot calmer now. I felt fluttering in the area where the IBS symptoms have usually been."

"I felt tingling in my arms. My left eye could see only purple light. At the same time, my right eye was seeing only the healer in white light. My eyes were shut throughout."

"I felt as though I had lit up to begin with and felt a little afraid but this passed about halfway through. Then I saw golden light with purple appearing in the middle. The turmoil within me, that I had arrived with, has now changed to a calmer feeling."

"I am feeling more positive now and there is tingling in my arms, shoulders and legs. I am quite surprised at my peace of mind throughout the session."

"I felt warmth throughout, except for my feet. I was aware of the colour lilac throughout. When the healer worked on my feet, I was aware of *lilac and green. When the healer worked on the hip to knee area, I felt blood flow through, which made my knee ache. My right eye has been a problem for two years. When the healer was working in that area, it was as though a sharp needle (that did not hurt) had pricked the right eye and it feels better now, as though it has cleared."*

"As an ex-nurse, I was paying attention to what was happening with my logical mind but I soon went with the relaxation. It felt as though my hands had raised by an inch and as though the healer had put my hands back down – but she had not done so." (Note: A medical student from the University of Birmingham was present and witnessed that the hands had not raised or been put back down.)

"I felt heat in the part where the pain was, and that pain is barely there now. When the healer touched my shoulders at the beginning, I felt tingles in my hands. Later, the healer touched my feet and I felt tingling in the base of my head."

"My shoulders feel freer and lighter. I feel really relaxed and a lot better. I am very pleasantly surprised and really chuffed. I can't believe how much better I feel now."

"I had felt concerned about my consultation with the doctor, but I feel better about it now. Bizarro! I didn't expect healing to work as well as it did. I felt tingling in my hands mostly and both arms. I loved it!"

* * *

I had suggested to all the patients, simply as a means of focusing their mind on something positive, that they imagine a golden-white light during the healing session. It is interesting that most of them saw purple instead; purple is the colour most strongly associated with healing. Regarding the "one week later" forms, the return rate was low, but on closer examination it became clear that some of the forms had not been posted. Nevertheless, enough forms came back to confirm that people were continuing to benefit from the previous week's healing session.

Out of the 192 patients in this second audit, 67 sent their feedback one week later. This was a high proportion, considering how many forms did not reach the patients.

The following comments add some interesting insights:

"I have felt a lot calmer and more peaceful since the healing session. I am not rushing around so much."

"I have benefited from the session for four weeks now. I am much less anxious."

"Before the healing session I felt terrible, but I was a different person afterwards. It was an amazing session."

"I am amazed that I still have no pain!"

"I have lost weight since the healing session but I am still smoking."

"I have not felt like myself in some situations, but every day my anxiety has been better. I have felt calmer and I am willing to try anything that will help."

"This treatment helped a lot with stress and sleeping."

"I have been more peaceful at home."

"I have been sleeping well for the past three weeks and have been feeling well in myself. Since the session, and having had one counselling session elsewhere, I have come on in leaps and bounds."

"There has been a positive effect since the healing session and, hopefully, this will get better. I do find healing very beneficial and would like regular sessions."

"I have felt more able to relax and more able to get problems into perspective. I would definitely like to have more sessions as I am sure that it can only bring more improvement."

"I feel that I can cope with situations a bit better now."

"This has been a journey of discovery for me and has made me more aware of other aspects of events and situations."

"Since the healing session, I have felt a lot more relaxed and have been able to sleep well most nights. However, I am still tired all the time and so I find it hard to concentrate well, although this has improved a lot."

"I have noticed a vast improvement since the healing session."

"After the session, the symptoms were less troublesome for a total of six days."

"After the first healing session, I felt good for a few days, but then the IBS started again."

"The one session I had was very uplifting and I feel that there has been some improvement."

"Since having this session, I have been constantly eating fruit. From having just one piece of fruit every two weeks, I am now having more than five per day. I felt very sick half an hour after the session, but since then I have had a constant craving for fruit every day. Monday this week, I just ate fruit all day. Before, I struggled to eat an apple once every two weeks. I would usually eat chocolate every day and, for a week after the session, I had not touched a piece. Usually, I would eat lots of chocolate every day, even when feeling unwell. I really think that the healing session has made this happen."

"Since the healing session, I have not been responding in my customary knee-jerk way to pressures placed upon me. I have actively sought measures to reduce stress and I feel better for it. Initially, I was sceptical but the session proved wholly worthwhile and points out things that a person does not always see."

• • •

Healers all around the world probably witness similar responses to those that fill my two audits. The difference is that many of the improvements described here have been witnessed by a senior consultant physician.

Another unusual aspect is that it is highly unlikely that any other healer has had the opportunity to give healing to people who had no prior intention of having any.

Added to this, few healers would be prepared to devise and complete the paperwork necessary to produce an audit. It took two and a half years to conduct the healing sessions involved in these two audits, and this part of the venture was a real pleasure; the administrative elements took many laborious hours, but it simply had to be done.

The results of the second audit provide almost identical results to the first. This correlation between the two further underpins the reliability of their respective findings. In research terms, "reliability" means that if the same exercise were to be repeated, we could expect similar results.

Anyone is welcome to use the primary data of these two audits for their own research purposes. I would simply ask that I be provided with any results, as it would be useful to link the studies together. Requests can be sent to me via my website.

After completing both of these audits, I continued to see patients as usual but I no longer documented their responses. Conducting an audit is a time-consuming business, and I felt that the results of 267 patients must surely be enough to pique the interest of medics, researchers and patients who are willing to enquire.

With the results of the audits being so impressive, I wanted to be able to give talks about these exciting findings, so I booked myself onto a course to learn how to produce slides and scripts for PowerPoint presentations.

Armed with my new skills, I was ready to put my graphs to good use, as you will find later.

Key Points

- A senior consultant physician witnessed his patients benefit from one 20-minute healing session, some to a remarkable degree.
- Few of these patients had accessed complementary therapies before, and almost all were highly sceptical that healing could help.
- These patients' symptoms were resistant to standard and specialist treatment, but they were helped in various ways by one session of spiritual healing.
- Figures 3, 4 and 5 reveal the placebo effect associated with compassionate care from a doctor (the grey columns), and the additional gains resulting from a healing session (the white columns).
- Patients with long-standing addictions were helped by one healing session.
- One healing session resulted in substantial improvements regarding pain relief, well-being, relaxation, relationships, energy levels and sleep quality.
- Improvements were retained for at least one week by almost all the patients who returned their "one week later" form.
- Patients who received healing were keen to have more.

- Patients who attended follow-up appointments months later confirmed that they had continued to benefit.
- Improvements for some may have been permanent.
- The two hospital audits – of 75 and 192 patients respectively – resulted in similar findings to each other, thereby confirming the reliability of both.
- Hardly any of these patients had received healing before and did not know what to expect, yet their comments reveal similar themes.

4

An Instant Recovery

D r Singh does not normally treat children, but a paediatrician who knew of his reputation asked if he would see a young teenager. The boy's symptoms continued to rage, despite all appropriate treatments with medication.

At his consultation with Dr Singh, the youth was in a great deal of pain, and there seemed to be no drug or treatment to alleviate his suffering. Dr Singh suggested that he have a healing session with me, and the boy – whom I shall call Joe – agreed.

Joe left his healing session completely free of pain and feeling elated. When he returned to his waiting mother he walked with a confident stride and a beaming smile. I saw the colour drain from her face when she saw him, and her jaw literally dropped. She was speechless. But, within a moment, she regained her wits and whisked him straight off for a blood test to have him checked out.

When I returned home that evening, the telephone was ringing. It was Joe. He told me that he had already tried calling me 15 times because he was so excited about the outcome of the healing session.

He admitted that, in the few strides from Dr Singh's room to mine, he had suddenly felt fear rising up within him. He realized that it was fear of the unknown, and he was gripped with worry about what might happen to him. However, I seem to have a knack for putting people at ease, and he confirmed that he soon relaxed once he was on the couch.

Dr Singh was keen to learn more about Joe's astounding recovery so he arranged to visit him at home a few weeks later. Joe and his mother agreed that their interview could be recorded. They gave permission for it to be shared with medical professionals and to be used in any other way that could help others.

A Grand Round is where doctors, surgeons and medical students gather in a lecture theatre on the hospital campus, and one of their number shares their new knowledge with the rest. When Dr Singh first presented this recording at a Grand Round, he invited me along. It must have been a surprise for the medics to hear a discourse that involved spiritual healing. It was clear to any listener that Joe was intelligent and, despite his young age, highly articulate. Hearing him speak directly to us in the audience had great impact.

To avoid repetition, the following transcript is an amalgamation of the tape recording and the written account that Joe provided on his experiences later.

Chest pain had been a problem for years but for about ten days prior to the hospital appointment, it had been a terrible burning sensation, going up and down all the time and made worse by eating. I had vomited several times, which badly hurt my throat, making it feel as though it was on fire. Several previous bouts had each lasted for two or three weeks but settled down with medication. Each bout seemed worse than the last one and really, really hurt.

I love school and sports but was unable to attend either. I had no energy to get up in the morning; I felt down and was unable to face the day. Eating only plain, bland food stopped the vomiting but did not help the symptoms.

When I saw the consultant (Dr Singh), I believed that only tablets and more medicine could help so when he suggested that I have a healing session, I thought the idea was rubbish and plain silly. I was in such a fragile state, though, that I was willing to do anything and thought "Well, it can't make me any worse," so I gave it a shot. In the few steps from the consultant's room to the healer's, I suddenly worried about what she was going to do to me, but I decided to try it anyway.

Sandy, the healer, made sure that I was comfortable on the couch and told me to close my eyes. When she asked me to imagine certain pictures in my mind, I wanted to laugh but stopped myself from taking the mick and decided to take it really seriously. I did exactly what she said. Throughout the session I felt relaxed and, towards the end, she guided my thoughts to imagining a happy future and feeling good about myself.

The burning in my chest was slightly better by the end, but it was still there. When Sandy said to open my eyes it felt as though I had been asleep, yet I knew for sure that I had been completely awake throughout. She asked if there was any pain still so I told her of the pain in my chest. She told me to close my eyes and imagine light shining into my chest and in 30 seconds or so it disappeared. I thought, "Is this a dream?" because the pain in my chest had really gone. Then I had a cramp in my right shoulder so I told Sandy, and we used the same technique on my arm and that pain went.

I have never liked having blood taken. I had to go for a blood test straight after the healing session and, as always, asked for the area to be numbed. But it was going to take 45 minutes and there wasn't time so, for the first time ever, I had to have blood taken without being numbed. I felt a sharp shooting pain so I closed my eyes and repeated the white light technique. The pain went in five seconds! I opened my eyes to see if the needle had been taken out but it was still in there. I thought, "This is wicked!" The nurse did not manage to get any blood from that vein so she had to do it again with a smaller needle. But I was not scared this time because I knew I could make the pain go away. It felt really cool to be able to do that.

That evening, I felt amazing – on top of the world. I wasn't stressing about anything; I felt happy and calm. We went out for a McDonald's to celebrate. On the way there, I had a headache so I asked Mom to turn the radio off and closed my eyes to imagine white light shining on my head. The headache went! Strange isn't the word! It felt wicked. When I think about it, it makes me feel happy in myself.

For the rest of the day after the healing session, I kept thinking "Did that really happen?" When I got home, I felt pleasantly tired and just wanted to relax.

Previously, I would be constantly worried that the pain would come back. In addition to that, I had always worried about stupid things, just like my mom does. When in school, I would think about the next lesson and check that I had done the homework, even though I knew that I had already done it. I always felt scared about homework. School projects would worry me loads. I would go around all my mates to see how many pages they had done to make sure I had done enough. But now, I know in myself that I've done what I should and I know that it's good work. I'm not worried about it any more.

Sandy gave me her Sleep Easy & Be Well CD and I listened to it every night for a week. Ever since then, though, I have been relaxed enough to fall asleep naturally.

Things that Sandy said have stuck in my mind and help me in day-to-day life. For instance, to relax any muscles whenever they might get tense; to imagine white light filling all the cells of my body; to understand that the past is gone and that the future will never come; that what will come, will come anyway so there's no need to worry about it.

I don't know what happened in the healing session and nor do I care! I am just amazed that I have no pain. It's just brilliant. I think my illness was caused by stressing about random stuff and it just built up and up.

Before the session, I didn't have much of a faith but, ever since, I've been asking my mom if we can go to church on a Sunday. We haven't got around to it yet but I've been meaning to go every single Sunday. I don't know why but it's as though I feel a bit closer to God. That might sound weird to other people, but you have to experience it for yourself to know what I mean.

Ever since that healing session, I have never felt better; I never stress any more and I always feel calm, relaxed and very happy.

I would recommend healing to anyone because it's so amazing.

• • •

Joe's mother also kindly took the time to write to Dr Singh about her observations and gave permission for me to reproduce her letter. This is what she had to say:

I didn't expect my son to benefit from the healing session except for perhaps some relaxation. Nothing prepared me for beaming smiles and colour in his cheeks! I was floored! I could not have believed it.

That first night I looked in on him, as I always do, and I had never seen him looking so rested, so asleep and so peaceful.

It's not just an improvement in his health; it's his whole character. He is so much more relaxed. I am still astonished at the phenomenal success of that healing session. My son experienced total and immediate relief from pain.

• • •

When Joe later came for a follow-up appointment with Dr Singh, I did not recognize him at all. Young teens change so quickly, and he was now tall, strong and confident. He snapped up the opportunity to have a healing session with me, but not because he was sick. He knew from experience that healing sessions are enjoyable, energizing and empowering.

Much later on, he attended a further and final appointment. Again, I did not recognize him. The last I heard – eight years later – Joe was still free of all symptoms. Dr Singh continues to play his recording at Grand Rounds and to cohorts of medical students.

• • •

Just one healing session changed Joe's life. However, most people need a series of weekly sessions before they notice substantial improvements. Other healers presumably experience similar variations with their own patients. Why the difference? If the healer is the same person, the healing energy could be expected to be reasonably constant, and therefore the only major variable must be the patient. There may be a difference within them that affects the level of healing that can be achieved. Joe, for example, was at the end of his tether. He had no other options left and he admits in his testimony that he surrendered himself to the process. My view is that this level of submission is key to achieving the greatest and swiftest healing results. If one person can reach that point, so can anyone else.

Key Points

- A complete and permanent recovery occurred within half an hour, despite the patient's extreme scepticism.
- Fear had been an underlying issue, causing persistent stress and worry.
- The symptoms disappeared along with underlying concerns.
- The patient had not realized how stressed he had previously been until after the healing session.
- A senior consultant physician and also a paediatrician were witness to the recovery.
- Individual cases like this will not convince the scientific and medical community that healing is beneficial, no matter how many there are.

5

Chasing the Research Grant

Two months after starting work at the hospital, I received an email from a fellow Healing Trust member that ignited a frisson of excitement. That morning, the National Lottery had announced that it was offering a total of £25,000,000 to charities and to the voluntary sector to conduct research programmes. The grants were specifically for health and social well-being projects that would normally be too difficult to find funding for. This certainly applied to healing.

The scientific and medical communities usually point to the lack of evidence in favour of complementary therapies, and contend that trials are often of poor quality. Nevertheless, the use of complementary therapies remains widespread with estimates that up to one in four people use them,[28] though this figure varies depending on how it is measured. Approximately £1.6 billion a year is spent by individuals on complementary treatments, and an NHS survey showed that during 1999 as many as five million patients consulted a CAM practitioner (Complementary and Alternative Medicine).

Among patients with gastrointestinal complaints, other surveys have estimated that as many as 50 per cent commonly use complementary therapies.[29] This high level of usage was in no way reflected by the hundreds of patients I saw at the hospital. All but a few told me that they had not tried a complementary therapy of any description. This does not mean that the official figures must be wrong; they will include countless numbers of gastro sufferers whose symptoms are not as extreme as those of the patients at Dr Singh's clinic.

Medical research councils, medical charities and drug companies are the main funders of medical research, but these organizations provide little support for the type of research we had in mind. Taken together, it has been estimated that they spend less than 0.01 per cent of their total budget on investigating complementary therapies. High-quality research is extremely expensive to conduct but, if research were to show that healing is beneficial to patients, a number of groups could gain from its use:

- Cost savings could be made by the NHS – and therefore taxpayers – if medication and surgery bills were found to be reduced.
- Businesses could gain financially by reduced sick leave payments. Furthermore, staff attending work regularly are likely to be more productive, and especially so if they feel well.
- With fewer people off work with long-term sickness, the government – and therefore taxpayers – could gain financially by reduced welfare payments.
- Individual members of the public may benefit – and therefore so might their families – in the many ways illustrated by the 267 patients included in my two audits and by the 200 patients involved in our trial.

• • •

However, not one of the above groups is likely to offer research funding for healing.

I took the news of the Lottery's announcement along with me to Dr Singh's clinic. It was made clear that this was a "one time only" opportunity. What were the chances of this occurring within the first weeks of my working with someone influential enough to do something about it?

Dr Singh agreed that this was a special opportunity that should not be allowed to pass by without a serious attempt to apply. Intrigued that healing seemed to be making a positive difference to his patients, he felt motivated to bring together the necessary parties to make an application.

The Lottery was aiming to fund:

> "... organizations that would produce and disseminate robust, research-based knowledge that will influence local and national policy and practice, to develop better services and interventions for people".

• • •

So far, so good – healing would meet the basic criterion of providing an intervention that could help people.

A condition of the grant was that a charity or voluntary organization must make the application and administer the programme. Dr Singh was a trustee of a medical charity called Freshwinds that provided integrated care to those with life-limiting illnesses. Their patients received spiritual healing and other complementary therapies alongside conventional medical care. Freshwinds were happy to take up Dr Singh's suggestion that they apply for the grant on our behalf.

It was strongly recommended that research professionals at a university or research facility should conduct the trial itself, as it is such a complex task. The Lottery was looking for projects that could stand up to peer review and be accepted for publication in scientific or medical journals.

Dr Singh approached a colleague at the University of Birmingham who had considerable research expertise relevant to our project. He was delighted when Lesley Roberts Ph.D. agreed to join the Steering Group. Another researcher from the University also joined, primarily to focus on a secondary element of the research, explained later. After the study had been completed, a statistician from the University would analyze the data. It was all coming together.

To my knowledge, no other Russell Group (UK) or Ivy League (USA) university – both known for world class research – had ever conducted a trial on spiritual healing. Having the University of Birmingham on board was a major achievement and very exciting.

To be able to conduct a clinical trial in the UK, a Primary Care Trust (PCT) needs to be involved. The PCT that governs Good Hope Hospital was the obvious contender as the healing work was anticipated to take place at Dr Singh's clinic.

Evidence had to be provided that the project was beneficial to members of the public, and that people wanted the project to take place. By this time, my first audit was well under way and already gave substantial data confirming both points. The final question on my "one week later" form asked if the patient would be interested in a series of six healing sessions, and Figure 12 shows that patients were overwhelmingly in favour.

For uniformity of the healing method and to ensure professional standards, I proposed that all of the healers involved must have been trained by the Healing Trust. In addition, they should be current members of the Healing Trust to guarantee that the healers would be subject to a strict Code of Conduct and disciplinary procedures. I also proposed that patients each receive a series of five or six weekly healing sessions.

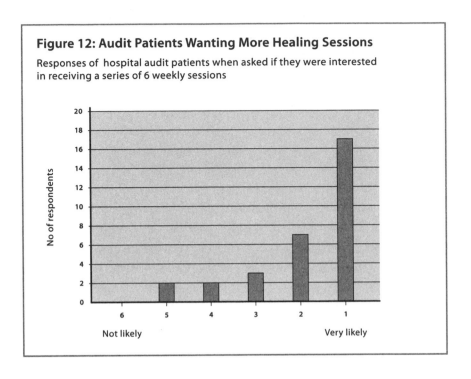

Figure 12: Audit Patients Wanting More Healing Sessions

Responses of hospital audit patients when asked if they were interested in receiving a series of 6 weekly sessions

. . .

The first Steering Group meeting between Freshwinds, the University researchers, Dr Singh and me was in January 2008 and we had much to discuss. A team of scientists was appointed by the Lottery to decide which applications should be awarded a grant. They were looking for randomized controlled trials (RCTs), the gold standard for research.

In an RCT, patients are randomly assigned to one of three groups. The first group receives the bona fide treatment, such as a real drug that is being tested. The second group receives a placebo, a fake version of the treatment, which might be a sugar pill. The third group receives no treatment at all, real or fake, and is called the "control" group. Scientists then endeavour to compare the results of the three different groups to establish whether the drug or treatment being trialled is effective.

For our trial, we needed a method of demonstrating that the positive effects were due to more than the placebo effect. If usual RCT procedures were followed, there would be trained healers giving treatment, and sham healers providing the placebo by mimicking a healer's actions. However, the practitioners and the actors would obviously both know which people were being treated by trained healers and which ones were not.

This immediately contravenes the conditions of an RCT, because it is imperative that nobody involved knows who is having the real treatment and who is having the sham. In addition, this method cannot be relied upon because every person has the natural potential to be a healer, trained or not. Accordingly, studies using sham healers have shown no difference between the so-called fakes and the trained healers.[30] In these trials the "bogus" and the "real" healing were equally beneficial, in comparison to the control groups, who had no treatment.

Our Steering Group decided that our researchers would devise a research protocol that did not employ sham healers.

A research protocol is the detailed description of how a programme will be conducted. It has to be precise in every detail so that other scientists can review the procedures and offer criticism if necessary. The aim is to develop a protocol that will produce results that can be relied upon. Also, if a future team of researchers wishes to conduct a similar trial, they can amend the same protocol to their needs. If their results are in keeping with the first trial, it helps to confirm the findings of both.

The subject of our research proposal was whether healing therapy, as an adjunct to conventional medicine, was beneficial for patients with IBS (irritable bowel syndrome) and IBD (inflammatory bowel disease). It is not known what causes these gastrointestinal disorders to develop in the first place. Both have unpredictable, embarrassing and painful symptoms that significantly affect almost every aspect of a sufferer's personal life. Physical health, psychological state, mobility, social life, sex life, work life and employment status are all adversely affected.[31]

Irritable bowel syndrome (IBS) is known to affect about 10 per cent of the population.[32] Common symptoms include abdominal pain, diarrhoea, constipation, bloating and erratic bowels. When investigated, blood tests, endoscopic investigation of the intestines and scans all give normal results. The cause of IBS is therefore a mystery, although it is thought to be due to psychological factors.

Inflammatory bowel disease (IBD) affects around one person in 1,000.[33] The term IBD covers two conditions – ulcerative colitis and Crohn's disease. Unlike IBS, these are diseases, where blood tests and endoscopic investigations disclose evidence of inflammation, and scans reveal abnormalities. However, it is not known why IBD develops in the first place. Both ulcerative colitis and Crohn's disease are intermittent, with weeks or months of mild or no problems, followed by periods of flare-ups. Outbreaks cause symptoms that can be excruciatingly painful and embarrassing. People with IBD are usually ill and miserable for a very long time.

Ulcerative colitis is a disease of the colon (the large intestine) that includes characteristic ulcers or open sores. The main symptom is usually constant diarrhoea mixed with blood, and abdominal pain.

Crohn's disease is an inflammatory disorder in which the body's immune system attacks the gastrointestinal tract. Common symptoms include recurring diarrhoea mixed with blood and mucus, abdominal pain, cramps, extreme tiredness and weight loss.

The persistent and fluctuating nature of both IBS and IBD means that patients need regular check-ups over a long period of time, thereby presenting high demands on healthcare resources.[34] No universally effective treatment exists for IBS or IBD, and options are limited. With so few conventional methods to help them, we thought these patients would surely be interested in any therapy that could help bring them some relief. It would be both fascinating and constructive to see whether healing could be of benefit in either or both of these two very distinct and distressing conditions. It was decided to use a variety of questionnaires. These would gather the maximum amount of data across all aspects of the particular ailments, as well as how the programme had affected their lives. Interviews with selected participants would add a further dimension. It would be impracticable and too complex to ascertain whether there had been an accompanying reduction in medication for these patients.

• • •

At last, in November 2009, we received the tremendous news that £205,000 had been granted for our project.

Congratulatory emails flew between the members of the Steering Group, and a press release was despatched.

I was invited to give talks at the Society for Psychical Research, the Doctor Healer Network, the Confederation of Healing Organisations, and the Royal Geographical Society. I delivered my newly produced PowerPoint presentation of the hospital audit graphs, culminating with the exciting news of the Lottery funding and information about the research programme. Broadcasting our success helped meet a condition laid down by the Lottery that we must publicize our award along with details of the project. The best coverage came when a BBC News programme came to the hospital to interview Dr Singh, one of his patients and me. The patient who agreed to be filmed had suffered for a long time with Crohn's disease. When asked by the reporter what she had to say about healing, she replied:

> *"Fantastic! I've had constant pain for nine years, literally crippled and brought to my knees. For four days after seeing Sandy, I didn't have a pain in my body at all. I thought I had died and gone to heaven!"*

When Dr Singh was filmed, he stated the following:

> *"We have seen benefits, sometimes unexplained and amazing benefits to some patients. [Yet] conventional scientific wisdom is that if you can't explain something then it can't be true."*

Key Points

- Applications for a Research Grant from the National Lottery had to be beneficial to the public.
- Successful applicants had to produce robust research that would be published in a scientific or medical journal and capable of influencing local and national policy and practice.
- Irritable bowel syndrome (IBS) affects at least 10 per cent of the population, and there is no medical cure.
- Inflammatory bowel disease (IBD) affects 0.1 per cent of the population, and there is no medical cure.
- Symptoms of IBS and IBD cause significant difficulties in all aspects of a sufferer's life.
- IBS and IBD patients usually suffer for many years.
- Depression often accompanies chronic medical conditions, including IBS and IBD.
- No universally effective treatment exists for either condition, and options are limited.
- An effective and affordable treatment for these patients would relieve pressure on NHS resources.

6

Existing Healing Research

To enable our grant application to be considered, a search of all related research first had to be made, to ensure that we were not repeating work that had already been completed or was in progress. Research has to extend the boundaries of what is already known.

Although the worldwide search of medical literature revealed no clinical trials of healing in IBS or IBD, it did find trials where healing had been found beneficial for other conditions.

Trials evaluating the effect of Therapeutic Touch – an American method of healing – in chronic pain sufferers found significant benefits in reducing pain and reducing the use of painkillers.[35] In other trials, healing had been found beneficial for osteoarthritis of the knee, burns patients and fibromyalgia.[36] Additional studies were found involving cancer, chronic pain, anxiety, wound healing and HIV. Each study concluded that healing had helped to reduce pain and anxiety, and had improved the patients' quality of life.[37]

Quality of life can be seriously impaired by medical treatments, and various studies have found that healing helps alleviate debilitating side effects. This is particularly the case for cancer treatments.

The majority of women who have had breast cancer are given hormonal treatment for five years. Side effects include hot flushes, aching joints, stress, anxiety, depression and lack of motivation. Understandably, a substantial number of patients seek respite by not taking the medication but this can diminish the long-term treatment benefits.

The University of Southampton (UK) conducted a trial using 12 women who were struggling with these side effects.[38] They were each given ten healing sessions by Healing Trust practitioners or equivalent. Not only were their symptoms alleviated, but they also spoke of feeling empowered and of experiencing a new serenity. Furthermore, they reported increased energy levels, enhanced well-being, emotional relaxation and re-engagement with their pre-cancer activities. These positive effects lasted between sessions and continued for varying lengths of time after completion of the course. One of the ladies admitted that she had previously been so badly affected by side effects that she had considered stopping her medication. Once she began having healing sessions, the symptoms were alleviated to such a degree that her intention to have a "drugs holiday" evaporated. In fact, while these women were receiving spiritual healing sessions, not one of them felt tempted to give up their hormonal treatment. This illustrates a valuable way in which healing can support conventional treatment.

There was no control group in the above study, but the positive outcomes demonstrated the safety and effectiveness of healing, and the results were significant enough to warrant controlled trials being conducted. With only 12 participants the trial was too tiny a sample size, in research terms, to achieve statistical confidence in its findings. However, it adds to the existing body of evidence, and scientists can group together any number of these small trials to look for patterns and trends on a grander scale. This method of research is called a review.

A review of healing trials that did include a control group –called a controlled trial – has been produced by David Hodges Ph.D. at the University of London. Among the many trials included, he typically found results such as the following examples:

- Healing on enzymes[39] and healing on stressed human blood[40] each produced positive results, despite the odds against this happening being less than 1 in 1,000.
- Healing on fungi and yeasts gave even greater significance – odds of 1.4 in 10,000 against the changes being due to chance.[41]
- Distant healing on fungal cultures gave a probability figure of less than 1 in 30,000.[42]
- A range of different trials on plants each gave a significance of less than 1 in 1,000.[43]
- Various trials on animals each gave a significance of less than 1 in 1,000 that the improvements seen were due to chance.[44]
- In human trials, a well-organized, double-blind study on wound healing, using non-contact healing, measured wound size on days 8 and 16. There were significant differences between experimental and control groups on both days.[45]
- A double-blind study was conducted on 96 hypertension patients. One group received distant healing and the other did not. Both

groups continued with their usual medical treatment. The results showed a significant improvement in the systolic blood pressure (when the heart contracts) of the group receiving healing, compared with the control group (although no significant changes in the diastolic blood pressure, when the heart is at rest and refilling with blood).[46]

In research terms, all of these results are termed "highly significant" or "very highly significant". Full details can be found on the Healing Trust's website.

• • •

The beneficial effect of healing on pain, anxiety and quality-of-life issues is complex and therefore difficult to measure. However, specialized questionnaires designed for the particular illness concerned have proved to be the most effective and reliable tool, and these were utilized in the following experiments:

1. A total of 60 volunteers suffering from tension headaches were split into two groups. The first group received a healing session, and the second group received sham healing. Pain relief was measured immediately after treatment and again four hours later using a specialized questionnaire. Results revealed a significant difference between the groups, with those who received healing reporting a 70 per cent reduction in pain.[47]

2. A total of 90 patients in a hospital cardiovascular unit suffering from anxiety were split into three matched groups. One received five minutes of healing, the second received five minutes of touch without healing, and the third received no touch or healing. The people receiving healing showed a highly significant reduction in anxiety following the treatment. They also showed significant anxiety reductions, compared with both the "touch without healing" and "no touch" groups.[48]

3. A total of 60 hospitalized cardiac patients suffering from anxiety were randomly assigned to one of two groups. The first received five-minute treatments of non-contact healing given by an experienced practitioner. The patients in the other group were given inexperienced practitioners who went through similar procedures but while doing mental arithmetic. Results showed

that the group receiving healing experienced a very significant reduction in anxiety.[49]

4. A double-blind, crossover study was conducted on the effect of distant healing on post-operative pain. Of people needing surgical removal of both impacted lower molar teeth, 21 were randomly assigned to control or treatment groups. The healers, located several miles away, concentrated on photographs of the patients. The resultant data showed a highly significant improvement in reduced pain levels as a result of the distant healing.[50]

• • •

All of the above experiments appear in greater detail in Hodges' review, along with many others. David Hodges and his colleague Tony Scofield Ph.D. conducted experiments of their own at the University of London. They soaked cress seeds in salt water to make it difficult for them to germinate and grow properly. Then, in nine different experiments, the gifted healer Geoff Boltwood held his hand over the treatment group seeds for just two minutes each. Over the next several days, the scientists photographed the treated and untreated seeds. The pictures offer visible evidence that the seeds given healing germinated sooner and grew substantially in comparison to the untreated seeds.[51]

Another experiment on plants was conducted in a commercial setting where a healer was asked to treat lettuce seeds before they were planted at an organic farm.[52] By the time the plants were ready to go to market, the lettuces that had received healing energy had yielded 10 per cent more crop than the others and had less slug and fungal damage. The researchers reached the obvious conclusion that there could be a commercial use for healing.

• • •

After having conducted research into various complementary therapies, Hodges and Scofield concluded that:

> If most complementary therapists were to recognize that they primarily harnessed healing energy and that the techniques ... they used were largely part of the ritual for achieving this, then complementary medicine would be in a much stronger position to defend itself from criticisms by conventionally trained scientists.

• • •

They also jointly produced a scientific paper that was published by the Royal Society of Medicine. Its conclusion states:

> Healing is ... largely viewed with scepticism by medical science, in spite of evidence that points strongly towards the need for an objective investigation and assessment of the phenomenon.
>
> If integrated into medical practice, [healing] could be a major advance in healthcare and potentially a significant factor in controlling medical costs.
>
> The mechanisms underlying healing appear to be radically different from those underpinning modern medicine.[53]

• • •

Experiments at the University of Connecticut further support these statements. A series of laboratory trials were conducted on human bone and tendon cells in Petri dishes.[54] The conclusion of a 2010 paper authored by Professor Gloria Gronowicz on these experiments states:

> ... Therapeutic Touch treatment of human bone cancer cell lines caused a significant decrease in matrix synthesis and mineralization, and differential effects on cell growth ... energy medicine may be beneficial to patients ... this technique ... has scientific validity and should be studied in more depth.

Gronowicz was surprised that healing did have an effect, and especially so to find that healthy cells grew faster and stronger, while cancerous cells became weaker.

• • •

Earlier laboratory experiments on human cells employed Matthew Manning, a well-known healer. In his book *The Healing Journey*, he describes giving healing to blood that had been mixed with saline solution. Normally, saline kills blood cells within five minutes. The cells given healing lived for 20 minutes – four times longer than the controls.

In other experiments, Matthew gave healing to cancer cells placed in liquid protein feed. Under these conditions, the death rate of cancer cells is usually 1,000 per millilitre of liquid. In 27 trials out of 30, the death rate of the cancer cells given healing increased by between 200 per cent and 1,200 per cent.

One of the scientists involved, William Braud Ph.D., described the results of Matthews's healing as "impressive". These and many other experiments are presented in Braud's book *Distant Mental Influence: Its Contributions to Science, Healing and Human Interactions.* As with Gronowicz's experiments, it was shown that healing improves healthy cells, yet simultaneously depletes cancerous cells.

• • •

A Japanese energy healing method called *johrei* was applied to different types of human cancer cells in vitro. In some, it was found that more cancer cells died in the samples given *johrei*. In others, the cancer cells that received *johrei* proliferated less than the controls.[55]

• • •

The National Health Service (UK) funded research at the University of Aberdeen to ascertain the effectiveness of spiritual healing in restricted neck movement.[56] A total of 68 patients received three healing sessions each, over a three-week period. Not only was neck movement in each direction significantly improved in comparison to the control group, but the severity of pain was also reduced. In addition, the treatment group significantly improved their scores for physical function, energy and vitality in comparison to the group that had not received healing.

• • •

Research aims to stretch the boundaries of knowledge and understanding, sometimes using different methods or by applying the same methods in a different context. Besides running a clinical trial, another means of conducting research is to undertake a "systematic review". This is where a research question is posed and then a review of all the research evidence relevant to that question is used to arrive at a conclusion. It is a method of combining all the available evidence and is regularly employed in healthcare. The Cochrane Collaboration, for instance, is a group of over 31,000 healthcare specialists in more than 120 countries who volunteer to routinely organize medical research information in this way. As a result, more informed choices can be made regarding the provision of care.

Another option is a "meta-analysis", where the statistics from different studies are contrasted and combined in the hope of identifying patterns or other interesting relationships. It is a mathematical technique that combines the results of individual studies to arrive at one overall measure of the effect of a treatment. Again, this method is often used to assess the clinical effectiveness of healthcare interventions.

Dr Daniel J. Benor, a Canadian medical doctor, has amassed a wealth of clinical trials, systematic reviews and meta-analyses regarding healing.[57] Of the extensive alphabetical list available on his website, the following selection is taken from the sections A to C. For ease of reading I have reworded some of the text.

1. A systematic review focused on the efficacy of distant healing involved a total of 2,774 patients.[58] A total of 23 randomized studies were reviewed – five with prayer healing, 11 with non-contact healing and seven miscellaneous distant healing approaches. A positive effect was found in 57 per cent of these. The authors concluded that "the evidence thus far warrants further study", which, in research terminology, means that the evidence has merit. One of its authors was Professor Edzard Ernst, the first Professor of Complementary Therapies in the UK.
2. A meta-analysis was conducted regarding the effect of healing on electrodermal activity (EDA).[59] This is a measure of electrical conductance of the skin, which varies depending on the amount of sweat-induced moisture present. When a threatening situation occurs, the "fight or flight" response is activated, which creates the tension needed to deal with the situation. One of the effects is instant sweat production, and this means that EDA reflects a person's state of anxiety. By attaching a meter to the patient's skin, it was found that healers could selectively lower and raise a patient's EDA. In a series of studies there were 323 sessions with four experimenters, 62 influencers and 271 subjects. Of the 15 studies, six (40 per cent) produced significant results. Of the 323 sessions, 57 per cent were successful.
3. A meta-analysis was conducted in 2000 regarding the effects of Therapeutic Touch on patients with anxiety.[60] A total of nine randomized studies were reviewed that met the criteria specified by the researchers. They concluded that Therapeutic Touch significantly reduced transient anxiety.

4. Using imaging technology, a study in 2005 demonstrated that sending thoughts at a distance correlates with the activation of certain brain functions in the recipients.[61] The recipient was placed in an MRI scanner and isolated from all forms of sensory contact from the healer. The healer then sent distant healing at random two-minute intervals that were unknown to the recipient. Very highly significant differences between experimental and control procedures were found. The researchers concluded that a healer can make an intentional connection with a person who has been isolated from the healer in every way, as this can be correlated to changes in brain function of the target individual.

5. A randomized control trial of healing was conducted that involved approximately 400 patients undergoing coronary artery bypass surgery at an American hospital.[62] There were three groups; one received healing, another received a visit, and the third was a control group that received neither. It was found that participants who received healing had a shorter hospital stay.

6. Double-blind preliminary studies were conducted to see if hands on healing affected enzyme activity.[63] Pepsin is an enzyme in the stomach that breaks down proteins and is therefore vital for digestion. A pepsin solution was added to egg albumen in test tubes, and measurements were made to track the level of protein breakdown. Prior to mixing, one test tube of enzyme was exposed to a healer's hands, a second to a non-healer's hands, and the third remained untreated. In all three trials the "healed" enzyme was found to have a significantly higher level of activity than the untreated control. These results suggest that healing aids digestion.

7. A study was conducted in order to determine whether healing could exert a beneficial effect on peak expiratory flow rates (PEFR) in people with asthma.[64] A total of 22 people with asthma each received healing for a ten-minute period. Their PEFR was found to improve significantly, and 18 of the subjects showed greater improvement a week later.

8. The following study involved only one patient, but the results were exceptional and mystified the researchers and medics.[65]

The patient's blood flow was blocked by clots, causing paralysis in the mid-chest level and below. The maximum improvement thought possible was to the level of three vertebrae lower in the chest. Treatment consisted of a 15-minute telephone call each day, followed by a distant energy healing session. Every three to four weeks there would be a three-day break. Recovery after five months reached the lower back. MRI and neurological examination confirmed that the subject had functionality almost to the base of the spine (L5/S1) and was continuing to improve.

9. A series of experiments was performed utilizing okra and courgette seeds germinated in acoustically shielded, thermally insulated, dark, humid growth chambers.[66] Healing energy was administered for 15 to 20 minutes every 12 hours, with the intention that the treated seeds would germinate faster than the untreated seeds. The objective marker was the number of seeds that sprouted out of groups of 25 seeds, counted every 12 hours over three days. Temperature and relative humidity inside the seed germination containers were monitored every 15 minutes. Healing energy had a very highly significant effect both compared with an untreated control and over time.

• • •

A number of medical doctors have written books that promote the use of healing alongside conventional treatment. Among them are Dr Deepak Chopra, Dr Andrew Weil and Dr Bernie Siegel, who have each produced inspirational bestsellers that are bursting with references to research trials from around the world.

Maxwell Cade was the first to work towards developing scientific equipment that could visually display brainwave changes during a healing session. Cade was a highly qualified British scientist who worked in radiation physics for the government and for industry. In 1976, he and Geoff Blundell developed a Mind Mirror.[67] This was an electro-encephalograph (EEG) that demonstrated the connection between healer and patient. Its screen revealed that, when giving healing, the healer's brainwaves quickly changed to low-frequency alpha waves. Alpha waves are linked with passive, meditative mental activity, the state associated with biological self-repair or homeostasis. Within moments of the healer beginning to work, the Mind Mirror showed that the patient's brainwaves entrained to the same alpha wave pattern as the healer's. This phenomenon was demonstrated at the Wrekin Trust 1978 Conference, held at the University of Loughborough, with an audience of 400 doctors, psychologists, scientists, healers and other professionals watching on closed circuit television.

Further tests by Cade involved placing the patient in a separate room from the healer so that no communication between them was possible, and nor could they see each other. An EEG was attached to each participant, and the patient had no idea when the healing would begin. Nevertheless, the EEG revealed the same entrainment within the patient, moments after the healer had begun to work. Cade's passion and enthusiasm was the driving force behind this investigative work; his sudden death in 1984 tragically marked the end of further research.

• • •

A more recent study in America confirmed that a person's positive healing thoughts have a noticeable impact on someone else's mind and body.[68] Dean Radin Ph.D. at the Institute of Noetic Sciences in California wanted to see if the partners of cancer patients could help their spouse by sending healing energy to them. The healthy partner attended a training course for three months in preparation for the trial. They were then directed to send healing at random periods chosen by a computer. The receiving partner relaxed in a distant, shielded room for 30 minutes, not knowing within which periods of time during this half-hour the healing would be sent.

The double-blind study ascertained that, overall, the skin conductance of the receivers increased during the periods that healing was sent. Increased skin conductance means that the skin has more sweat, the production of which is stimulated by the sympathetic nervous system. Sweating is an indication of psychological or physiological arousal. Therefore, measuring skin conductance can identify changes in a person's state of nervousness or calm. These patients also described experiencing a warm feeling inside. This sensation mirrors the comments that patients often make about healing. However, the study was not designed to discover whether these responses actually promoted healing in any way.

• • •

Though not conducted in laboratory conditions, probably the most dramatic example of absent healing in action is the story of Dr Hew Len. Over 30 years ago, he began work as a clinical psychologist at the Hawaii State Hospital. His clinic was a special ward specifically for mentally ill criminals who had committed extremely serious crimes. They were so dangerous that they were permanently shackled and never allowed outside. No day passed without an attack on a fellow inmate or on a member of staff. Up until the arrival of Hew Len, previous appointees to his post had not stayed much longer than a month, and staff members were often off sick with stress.

When he arrived, instead of seeing any patients, he quietly viewed their files and photographs in his office and then conducted a Hawaiian method of distant healing in his mind. As time went by, the patients began to improve. Medications were reduced, and some inmates were allowed outside, no longer shackled. Staff absence dwindled. In less than four years, all but a few of the prisoners had been released. The last few were sent elsewhere, and the secure unit was closed down.[69]

Hew Len's example points to the value of sending healing to perpetrators of crime. It is natural for us to feel empathy for victims, but if we also send healing to offenders there may be fewer victims in the future. And with the obvious advantage of healers not needing to be in close proximity to offenders, or to require their permission, the scope is limitless. Prior permission is not required for absent healing, in much the same way that prayers are said for people without their knowledge or consent.

It may seem impossible that distant healing could be effective, but the work of Cade and those who came after him seems no less outlandish than what quantum physicists term "entanglement". This is something observed in subatomic particles called quarks – if quarks with identical spin are paired and separated, changing the spin on one will instantaneously change the spin of its partner, regardless of how many miles apart they are. And of course, atoms are the building blocks of the cells that make up our physical bodies. Surely we must be subject to the same effect in some subtle way?

The work of physicist Amit Goswami seems to demonstrate this. In an experiment, Goswami had two people meditate together, then placed them in two separate chambers that were electromagnetically impervious. It was impossible for them to see or hear each other, or make contact in any way. He then repeatedly flashed a light near one person's eye, causing the firing of a certain frequency in the brain. At the same moment, the other person's brain fired similarly, even though that person could not possibly see the light.

• • •

Whatever the reality is, I choose to believe that healing energy is working at this quantum level. When sending distant healing (as well as in-person healing) I imagine my patients being illuminated with brilliant light that is charging them with positive energy and elation.

• • •

Those who are not shocked when they first come across quantum theory cannot possibly have understood it.

Niels Bohr [70]

I think I can safely say that nobody understands quantum mechanics.

Richard Feynman [71]

• • •

Judging from all of the above, it would seem that quantum physicists ought to have less difficulty accepting that beneficial healing energies exist than conventional scientists might. Throughout history, the scientific community has found it very difficult to accept a new paradigm that contradicts established knowledge.

• • •

Bruce Lipton Ph.D. was a cell biologist and professor at the National Institutes of Health, USA, and he maintains that positive emotion is a necessity for physical health. In his book *The Biology of Belief,* he writes about the chemical activity that is visible at cell level and how he discovered that too much negative emotion tips the balance of health within the cell. He explains that health is, of course, supported by diet and exercise but that it is also affected by stress and optimism.

Lipton says that the main thing that influences the cells of our body is our blood. If we see someone we dearly love, our perception causes a release into the blood of oxytocin, dopamine and hormones that encourage the growth and health of cells. Conversely, seeing something frightening releases stress hormones – cortisol, histamine, norepinephrine – which put the cells on alert and into a protection mode. Worry, stress and other negative emotions all have the same effect. If these emotions persist, Lipton contends, the imbalance can eventually develop into an illness or disorder. People usually comment on how uplifting healing feels, and Lipton's work indicates that the brighter state of mind they experience causes a physical contribution towards the health of their cells.

• • •

Academics who believe that healing should be further researched include Professor Peter Fenwick, a consultant neuropsychiatrist at King's College London. He has studied the phenomenon of healing and says:

> There are four possibilities. Either we are dealing with fraud on a massive scale; or large numbers of able and gifted researchers are simply wrong; or hundreds of reports disproving healing have not been published. All these seem unlikely, so we're left with the possibility that the effect is real.[72]

• • •

Professor Harald Walach, a psychologist at the University of Northampton, is quoted as saying:

> We should take this phenomenon seriously even if we don't understand it. To ignore it would be unscientific. Our work shows that there is a significant effect, and despite it being the most widely practised alternative remedy, science has only recently begun to investigate whether spiritual healing actually works. Scientists and doctors simply assumed that it didn't.

• • •

In answer to critics who say that much healing research is flawed and that any effects are due to the placebo effect, the Confederation of Healing Organisations (CHO) commissioned the University of Northampton to produce the largest ever meta-analysis of non-contact healing.[73]

It focused on two separate groups, the first being only plants, animals and cell cultures, so that the placebo effect could be discounted. The second group included only humans. The researchers excluded any studies that did not meet their standards, yet the results remained significant for both groups. Professor Paul Dieppe of the University of Exeter commented on the findings thus:

> *This is a rigorous, high-quality scientific report, and it clearly shows that healing intention can have beneficial effects on living systems, both human and non-human.*

In this study, the scientists found that it made little difference if they excluded all of the trials that fell below their standards of methodological excellence. This suggests that those trials that were below par did actually demonstrate that healing was effective; it was only because their methodology could be criticized that they were disqualified from the meta-analysis.

To help future investigators to steer clear of such pitfalls, their work includes a section giving comprehensive guidance. However, for scientists to be able to investigate healing, they need financial backing, and they also need to know that they will not be ridiculed and ostracized by the scientific community.

Professor David Peters of the University of Westminster has this to say about the findings of existing research:

> *Science now supports some of the key principles of traditional healing – that the body and mind are effectively inseparable; that the body–mind has untapped and inbuilt healing responses; that complex systems are self-sustaining because a flow of information organizes them.*[74]

• • •

At the time of the CHO's meta-analysis being published, our own research paper was on the verge of being sent to a medical journal. Academically, we hoped that we would be adding yet another piece of convincing evidence to the existing mass. In practical terms, I hoped that the positive results would persuade medics and patients alike that healing really does make a difference. Positive results might then take us a step closer towards my ultimate goal – having healing made available to the British public via the NHS.

Key Points

- Extensive research shows the following:
  - Healing is effective for people in respect of a wide range of issues, including physical, mental and emotional problems.
  - Healing is effective on animals and plants, and on human cells in Petri dishes.
- Healing on human cells in Petri dishes strengthens healthy cells and, at the same time, depletes cancer cells.
- The results of healing on animals, plants and cells in vitro demonstrate that the placebo effect cannot be a factor.
- Distant healing is effective.
- When distant healing is sent without the knowledge of the recipient and has been effective, the placebo effect cannot be a factor.
- Healing supports medical treatments by reducing side effects.
- Healing supports surgical procedures by alleviating distress beforehand and by speeding recovery afterwards.

7

The Research Programme

Soon after hearing the terrific news that we had been awarded a grant, our Steering Group met to begin getting the project under way.

The main priority for the researchers was to finalize the study protocol; they had to design a carefully structured, written plan to ensure that the programme ran smoothly to a successful conclusion. It had to be robust enough to withstand peer review in order to validate the systems and procedures used. Questionnaires, an information booklet for participants, letters and forms all had to be devised and finalized. Only when all of this documentation was completed could ethics approval be applied for.

Whenever research involves interviewing people, giving them questionnaires, accessing their medical records or offering them a treatment, ethics approval is mandatory. This is to ensure that participants are treated with respect, are informed about the research, have given their consent and are not harmed in any way by the treatment.

Another priority was setting up detailed, official partnership agreements between Freshwinds, the University of Birmingham and the Primary Care Trust. Each organization needed to commit to devoting specific resources to the project, which included personnel, office space, treatment rooms and any other elements involved.

Healers had to be recruited, too. I was most surprised to learn that the healers would be paid for their work as I had anticipated that we would be seeing the patients in a voluntary capacity; but, of course, it made sense that the employment of healers should be on a formal and professional basis.

All the participants were to be recruited from Dr Singh's outpatients clinic. At their usual consultation with him, or with one of his colleagues, each suitable IBS and IBD patient was asked if they would like to be involved in the project. If they agreed, they were immediately given an appointment with the research assistant, who provided them with information to share with their families before making a decision.

Once their consent had been received, the patients were randomized between two groups, with equal numbers of IBS and IBD patients in each. The "Intervention Group" patients would then embark upon a series of five weekly healing sessions, but the "Waiting List Control Group" would not receive treatment until 12 weeks later. That way, the results of the Intervention Group (those who received the treatment immediately) could be compared at Week 6 and Week 12 with the Waiting List Group, before the latter began receiving healing sessions.

The first questionnaires were to be completed at Week 0 – before the healing sessions began – and then repeated at Week 6, Week 12 and Week 24. Given that the Intervention Group received healing immediately and the other group did not, direct comparisons could be made between them until Week 12. After this, the Waiting List Group would begin to have healing sessions, which means the Intervention Group's Week 24 would not have a control group to compare against. Instead, this Week 24 data would establish whether any benefits identified at the previous stages had been sustained.

One would think that it could be useful to compare the results of the patients on our trial with those who had refused to take part. There may be a difference between those who are willing to try a safe but strange approach and those who are not. However, this is against standard research protocol; only people who are prepared to be randomized can be included, which means that they must be prepared to have the treatment if they are chosen for that group. Therefore, people who are *only* prepared to be in the control group – the group that receives no treatment at all – cannot be accepted. This means, of course, that only people willing to have healing were included in the trial, thereby making the participants "selective". Ideally, research trials require "non-selective" participants, picked totally at random so there is no bias. However, this is impossible for any trials involving human beings because people have to agree to take part.

To gather information, each participant completed three different questionnaires. Everyone on the programme completed a general questionnaire called MYMOP, described later, plus two others that were specifically intended for their particular condition. Thus, the IBS people completed a different set from those for the IBD patients, but both groups completed MYMOP.

All of the questionnaires employed had previously been widely used in clinical research and were validated. Validation means that these forms have been rigorously assessed to confirm their reliability, validity, reproducibility and responsiveness. This ensures that the questions are detailed and precise enough to avoid ambiguity and are able to register changes in a patient's condition. Thus, the data gained can be expected to provide meaningful and useful information.

Together, the various questionnaires used would establish whether healing benefited patients in measurable ways, and also how they felt within themselves throughout the course of the programme. A small number of patients were also invited to in-depth interviews to get a fuller picture of how the treatment had affected their lives.

Researchers talk of quantitative data and qualitative data. As the words suggest, one refers to quantities and the other to qualities. Quantities can be measured and weighed whereas qualities are sensed and perceived. Measured and weighed quantities can be thought of as solid, whereas perceived qualities can be thought of as soft. Quantitative data would therefore be the equivalent of the bare bones or skeleton, and qualitative data would be the flesh that brings those bones to life.[75] Qualitative, "flesh" data aims to discover the human elements that affect a person's life. With both types of data to work with, a clearer picture can be gained that brings real meaning to research results. In our study, the questionnaires would provide the quantitative data regarding quality of life and symptoms. The subsequent interviews with selected patients would add qualitative data by discovering their personal perspectives on their experience.

The MYMOP questionnaire – Measure Yourself Medical Outcomes Profile – was completed by all participants. This was created by Dr Charlotte Paterson, a GP (general practitioner) from Somerset who has made complementary therapies available to her patients for many years.

Published studies have shown that MYMOP is practical, reliable and sensitive to any changes in the patient's condition. It has been extensively used in clinical research and is a validated instrument, designed to gather highly individualized information that is particularly patient-centred.

The MYMOP questionnaire is brief, which increases its feasibility and acceptability, thereby leading to high response and completion rates. Its simple structure and straightforward scoring make it easy to chart the scores of individual patients over a period of time.

MYMOP aims to measure the outcomes that the patient considers to be the most important. The patient chooses one or two symptoms that are causing them the worst difficulty and for which they would like the most help. Then they choose an activity of daily living that they cannot do or cannot manage properly because of this symptom. These choices are written down in the patient's own words, and the patient then scores them for severity over the previous week. On each follow-up questionnaire, the wording of the chosen issues remains unchanged, and the patient scores them afresh.

All of these scores are added together to get a final figure and, in our study, the final figures for Week 0, Week 6, Week 12 and Week 24 would reveal a picture of the outcome. Week 0 questionnaires were completed before the first healing session, giving what is called the "baseline", against which the subsequent figures would be compared.

As well as MYMOP, the IBS patients completed a widely used and validated questionnaire called IBS-QoL (Irritable Bowel Syndrome Quality of Life). This was developed by a team of researchers at the University of Washington in Seattle. Its questions cover eight specific areas of a person's life – feeling unwell or unhappy, daily life activities, body image, health, worry, food avoidance, social reaction, and sexual/relationship aspects. It also evaluates bowel issues and the body as a whole. The individual gives a score for each particular issue, ranging from scoring just one point for "not at all" through to five points for "extremely". These scores are added together and then averaged for a total figure, higher scores indicating a better quality of life. The IBS-QoL was designed to be completed by the patient and takes about ten minutes.

In addition to the MYMOP and IBS-QoL questionnaires, the IBS patients also completed the Birmingham IBS questionnaire. This was developed at the University of Birmingham to ascertain the severity of IBS symptoms. Its questions ask how frequent and intense their physical problems had been over the previous four weeks.

All of the people with IBD completed a MYMOP and also an IBDQ (Inflammatory Bowel Disease Questionnaire). The IBDQ was developed at McMaster University, Ontario, by a team of researchers who discovered that almost 50 per cent of IBD patients under-reported the various difficulties they experienced unless they were encouraged by a reminder list. Until this in-depth investigation, their doctors and even spouses had not realized the full extent of their suffering. The IBDQ is a respected quality of life questionnaire used extensively in academic research and clinical trials.

The inflammatory bowel disease (IBD) group was originally to be populated only by patients with ulcerative colitis, but there were too few patients with this condition. It was therefore decided to recruit people with Crohn's disease to reach our goal of 100 in the IBD group.

Ulcerative colitis patients completed a Simple Clinical Colitis Activity Index (SCCAI) questionnaire. This was jointly authored by researchers at the Royal Free Hospital School of Medicine in London and the Queen Elizabeth Hospital in Birmingham (UK), to help doctors evaluate the severity of colitis in an accurate and easy way. This questionnaire would be useful to reveal any changes in symptoms during our programme.

Those with Crohn's disease completed a modified version of the Harvey-Bradshaw Index questionnaire. This consists of just five questions relevant to Crohn's symptoms.

Every participant therefore completed three questionnaires at each of the four stages – Week 0, Week 6, Week 12 and Week 24. If none of the 200 participants quit the programme, there would be a total of 2,400 questionnaires to process and evaluate. Armed with this amount of data, our researchers and statisticians should have a wealth of information from which to produce meaningful results.

• • •

The healers were not involved with the questionnaires. Our only remit was to deliver healing sessions.

Although the healers employed on the research programme were all using the same method of healing, we were allowed to help the patients relax beforehand in our own individual way. Some healers simply instruct the patient to take a few deep breaths.

I use this method if talking might disturb others, such as at our healing centre where a number of people could be receiving healing in the same room. If I am alone with the patient, as at the hospital, I use a short and simple visualization that gives the patient a useful technique to take home with them.

• • •

My final healing session on the programme, which was the last one of the entire project, was in June 2012. Once this patient's Week 24 questionnaire arrived, the researchers and statisticians would be able to conclude processing the mountain of data and reveal the outcomes.

Key Points

- NHS patients were to be recruited who continued to have IBS/IBD symptoms despite treatment by their GP (general practitioner) and specialist medical care.
- The main questionnaire (MYMOP) would determine whether people's lives had improved, not whether issues relating to IBS or IBD had been alleviated.
- The second questionnaire would determine whether people's lives had improved in respect of the specific difficulties caused by IBS or IBD symptoms.
- The third questionnaire would determine whether the physical symptoms of IBS or IBD had been alleviated.
- A small selection of patients would be interviewed to gain their personal perspectives.
- Comparisons were to be made between the Intervention Group and Waiting List Control Group at Week 6 and Week 12 to see if the group that received healing gained more than the group that did not.
- The Intervention Group's Week 24 figures would reveal whether benefits were retained in the longer term (19 weeks after their final session).

8

The Results

The unconventional subject matter of our study was likely to be a magnet for denigration, academic and otherwise. The Steering Group and the University's executive were bound to be alert to these risks, and would have aimed to minimize the possibility of criticism. Our researchers had their own professional reputations to protect as well as that of the University, which, as a member of the Russell Group, takes pride in being known for first-rate research.

Going on the range of positive patient responses that we had personally witnessed when seeing our patients, the other two main healers and I felt optimistic that the research results should be impressive. However, a great deal can depend on how researchers manipulate and present data, and this can be affected by their beliefs and attitudes. If researchers are biased, either in favour or against the subject of a trial, then the presentation of the results can be slanted accordingly.

But I had no doubt that the researchers on our Steering Group would present the results fairly. Nevertheless, I suppressed any dreams of triumph. It seemed to me that the outcome of a research programme could be like a court case where, despite evidence pointing to a defendant's innocence, they are found guilty, or vice versa. Perhaps that is why a research programme is called a "trial".

Another similarity between a research project and a court case is that all of the information involved has to remain totally confidential until it has been officially revealed. Prior disclosure of research findings could undermine confidence in them. Worse, if a research paper's robustness is disputed prior to its publication, an academic journal may not be prepared to print it at all.

At last, the meeting to present the findings arrived. Until then, the Steering Group had been given no hint as to how the incoming data was panning out. Five years had gone by since I had first approached Dr Singh about applying for the grant; this would be the moment when we would know whether our efforts had been at all worthwhile.

In short, looking at all of the numbers and graphs being shown to us, it was clear to me that healing had indeed made a significant difference. Dr Singh and I were exultant.

One of the graphs seemed to show that the Control Group had benefited slightly while they were waiting for their healing sessions to begin. I learned that this is a common feature of trials involving human beings. Even when people know that they are taking a sugar pill and are told categorically that it cannot do them any good, they often still improve. But in our study, the participants had not even started getting their "sugar pill" – in this case, their healing sessions. Their positive response may be due to the Hawthorne effect – described earlier – where patients improve when they feel that someone is taking an interest in their plight.

Although the Control Group in our trial improved by a small degree while they were waiting, the people who received healing sessions showed considerable improvements by comparison. Furthermore, the gains they reported followed a similar pattern to those in my audits.

Knowing that our study had been a success for healing was very exciting, but I was unable to share the cause of my elation with anyone outside of the Steering Group. Strict confidentiality was necessary until the research papers had been officially published, which would be a very long while as all co-authors must contribute their part and then agree to the wording of the final draft. The paper then has to be sent for peer review to academics within the originating university who were not involved in the trial. Any feedback is then considered and dealt with until a document agreeable to everyone is finalized.

Once the text of a research paper has been agreed, the authors can approach a scientific journal to ask if they will publish it. Naturally the most prestigious appropriate journal is the first one to ask. The accepting journal then sends the research paper to its own choice of independent academics and, again, it is scrutinized for the legitimacy of its content and process. Any feedback is forwarded to the editor of the journal, who conveys it back to the authors. If the journal is satisfied, it is scheduled to fit into an upcoming volume and goes to print.

Across both IBS and IBD, the baseline data at Week 0 revealed that it was the physical symptoms that caused patients the most concern. The main sources of distress were pain and problematic bowel activity, which – unsurprisingly – had a significant impact on patients' physical activity in their work life, social life and sex life and made them feel utterly miserable. The results that follow give an indication of how spiritual healing improved their situation.

Quantitative Results

This section includes the official findings of the research trial along with my own supplementary comments and analysis. I have tried to make it clear when a statement is mine rather than taken from the published research paper.[76] In the event of doubt, viewing the paper itself will clarify.

For ease of reading, the results of the trial are reported here without the technical jargon and fine detail needed to satisfy a medical researcher. The academic paper itself is the obvious source of such data, for those who wish to refer to it. Any numerical scores quoted are taken from the tables that appear in the research paper. The tables themselves are far too complex to be worth reproducing here.

My interpretation of the score improvements expresses greater benefit to the patients than the research paper conveys. The researchers aimed to be cautious in how they reported the results, and perhaps this explains the difference. To substantiate my explanations and statements, I have taken care to underpin them by referencing a reliable source

Where I have used the word "significant" in this chapter, it means significant in research terms and mirrors a statement in the research paper. "Statistical significance" conveys change in mathematical terms – the odds against the outcome happening by chance. "Clinical significance" reports the meaning – the difference it makes to a patient's life.

In trials, it is important to distinguish between statistical and clinical significance because a treatment might be statistically significant but not improve the patient's quality of life. In our study, the measurements used to establish whether the therapy was effective or not were provided by the patients themselves. The questions were focused on the patients' symptoms and their ability to lead a normal life. On the face of it, then, a significant statistical improvement in our trial ought to mean that there had been a corresponding clinically significant improvement.

Statisticians and researchers produce an array of different figures to convey results, and I have endeavoured to present their findings clearly and precisely. Should my additional interpretation of the findings raise queries, the paper itself is publicly available for clarification.

As each person gave their consent to be part of the programme, they were randomly assigned to either the "Intervention Group" or to the "Waiting List Control Group". Both groups completed their first set of questionnaires at Week 0 to gather baseline information about their current state of health and quality of life.

The Intervention Group then embarked upon five healing sessions, ideally every week. At Week 6 they completed a second set of the exact same questionnaires to see if any changes had occurred. At the time of completing the Week 6 questionnaires, 42 per cent of the Intervention Group had not yet received all five sessions, perhaps because of their holiday arrangements or other commitments. Therefore, one or two sessions for almost half of the Intervention Group took place after they had completed their Week 6 questionnaires. The Week 6 figures would reveal whether healing had made a difference to their physical symptoms and to their lives, whether or not they had yet received all five sessions.

In total, 78 per cent of the Intervention Group ultimately attended all five sessions well before Week 12. At Week 12, they completed another set of the same questionnaires to see whether the measures noted at Week 6 had changed. The people allocated to the Waiting List Control Group received no healing for the first 12 weeks while they completed their respective sets of Week 0, Week 6 and Week 12 questionnaires. This "control" data would then be contrasted against that of the Intervention Group. After they had completed their Week 12 paperwork, they were able to start their series of five healing sessions, most likely beginning at Week 13.

Normally, a control group would not receive the treatment being investigated, but it would have been unfair to deny our patients the opportunity to have healing. They had certainly been willing to have sessions, because they were prepared to be allocated to the Intervention Group when they first signed up. Indeed, when they were called for their healing appointments three months on, they followed the same pattern of high attendance and low drop-out as the Intervention Group. Once they had received their series of healing sessions, their Week 24 results could again be compared with those of the Intervention Group. To convey their dual role in the programme they were called the Waiting List Control Group in the research paper, instead of simply the "control group".

Both the Intervention Group and the Waiting List Control Group completed their final set of questionnaires at Week 24. For the Intervention Group, this was 19 weeks after their final healing session and would reveal whether any benefits had been retained in the longer term. The Waiting List Control Group did not begin their healing sessions until after Week 12, so their Week 24 was only seven weeks after their final session.

Figure 13 makes it easier to understand that the Intervention Group's Week 12 results and the Waiting List Control Group's Week 24 results are both seven weeks after their final session. Thus, the results for these two questionnaire time points could be expected to be similar to each other.

One could also suppose that the Week 24 figure for the Intervention Group might be lower than any other figures because their Week 24 was 19 weeks after their final session and any gains might have reduced by then. Both of these suppositions will be discussed in detail later.

Figure 13: Timetable of Healing Sessions & Questionnaires

Table showing when each group received healing and when they completed questionnaires

H Scheduled Healing Sessions. In practice, sessions for some patients were spread over a longer period. Others did not complete the sessions.

Q Questionnaires completed at Weeks 0, 6, 12 and 24.

Q Questionnaires completed seven weeks after the final healing session for each group.

Week No.	0	1	2	3	4	5	6	7	8	9	10	11	12	13	14	15	16	17	18	19	20	21	22	23	24
Intervention Group	Q	H	H	H	H	H	Q						Q												Q
Waiting List Group	Q						Q						Q	H	H	H	H	H							Q

Having now set the parameters of the study and explained some of the terms and terminology, we can turn to the actual results.

Quality of Life (MYMOP)

The primary goal of the research trial was to see if healing improved lives, and the main tool chosen to measure this was the MYMOP questionnaire. As described earlier, MYMOP is centred around the patient's experience of life, not whether they have recovered from specific ailments. It aims to discover what is troubling a patient the most and determine whether the treatment under investigation is bringing about improvements. Patients are asked to describe their two worst symptoms and then identify activities that are hindered by them. Using a seven-point scale, patients give a score for each symptom and for each activity so that any changes can be measured. In our trial, we might expect bowel problems to be identified as the worst problem, but it could be something else entirely.

All participants, whether they had IBS or IBD, completed this questionnaire. As one might guess, patients identified physical difficulties as being the most problematic for them. Pain was one of the two worst symptoms for 25 per cent of the participants. "Bowel habit" was one of the worst for 17 per cent of cases, and other common problems were diarrhoea, cramps and bloating. Whatever their worst two symptoms were, these had been making it difficult for patients to go to work, exercise and socialize, in varying degrees. With these elements being the prime activities of a normal day, it is no surprise that their quality of life had been seriously impaired.

The group that received healing from the outset – the Intervention Group – gained a significant improvement for each of their two worst symptoms and also for activities at Week 6 (all at either $p<0.001$ or $p=0.001$). These significant gains were maintained to Week 12 (all at either $p<0.001$ or $p=0.001$) and to Week 24 (all at $p<0.001$ or $p=0.001$).

This table explains the meaning of the statistical results that follow:

Probability

$p=0.05$ means odds of one in 20 (statistically significant)

$p=0.001$ means odds of one in 1,000 (highly significant)

$p=0.0001$ odds of one in 10,000 (very highly significant)

The phrase "$p<0.05$" means that the probability that the difference between the treatment group and the control group is due to chance is less than one in 20. (To arrive at this figure, divide one by 0.05.) Thus, the smaller the probability numbers, the less likely that the change is due to chance.

In medical research, $p=0.05$ (one in 20) is usually accepted as being significant[77] but, at the planning stage, the University researchers had raised the bar for our trial. They specified that $p<0.005$ (less than one in 200) would denote significance in respect of "sub-scales and domains", which translates to "symptoms and activities" within the MYMOP questionnaire. With results of $p<0.001$, the statistical significance in our trial for symptoms and activities were five times better than the raised bar, and 50 times better than the level normally accepted for medical research.

As is often the case in clinical trials, the Waiting List Control Group improved slightly even though they had not received the treatment. But even when compared against this slight improvement, the results for the Intervention Group still remained at the same level of significance for each of their two worst symptoms and for activities at Week 6, and at Week 12 (all at p<0.001).

Probability figures convey the "statistical significance" of how unlikely it is that the results obtained are due to chance. In trials, they may give no indication of the magnitude of the difference. "Clinical significance" is more meaningful to the patient, because it conveys the practical importance of a treatment – it reports a genuine, palpable and noticeable effect on daily life. Clinical effects are expressed by a change in score, the extent of which indicates the amount of change that took place.

Using MYMOP, a decrease in score denotes an improvement, with a drop of one unit meaning that an individual has probably improved by a noticeable degree. Thus, the larger the decrease in score the greater the positive clinical significance.

Taking the MYMOP figures for the IBS and IBD groups together as a whole, changes to their two main health problems had been scored along with the activities affected by them. As mentioned earlier, the scores referred to here are taken from the table that appears in the research paper.

At baseline (Week 0), the two worst symptoms and the affected activities were each scored at four units by the Intervention Group and by the Waiting List Control Group. By Week 6, the scores for the Intervention Group had each decreased by one unit (from four down to three), indicating a clinically determinable improvement. At Week 12, the score decreased again by a further one unit, from three down to two. For us healers, it was exciting to have scientific confirmation that our work improves lives to such a tangible degree.

The additional decrease in score by Week 12 could only be due to one of two things, or a combination of both.

One possibility could be in respect of the 42 per cent who had not received all five of their sessions before completing the Week 6 questionnaire. These people received their last one or two sessions after Week 6. The benefits gained from these later sessions could be the cause of the further decrease in score at Week 12. If so, then it would mean that additional benefits occurred through having those additional healing sessions. The other possibility is that people continued to improve after their final healing session. Either way, receiving healing sessions caused improvements to take place.

Given that Week 12 was at least one month after their final healing session, one might assume that some initial gains could have diminished by the time patients completed that questionnaire. Taking this into account, the Week 12 scores are even more impressive than they first seem.

One might also suppose that the Week 24 figures for the Intervention Group might be worse than earlier scores, because this questionnaire was completed 19 weeks after their final session, and gains could have reduced by then. Indeed, the two worst symptoms and also activities were each scored at three, one unit higher than they had gained by Week 12, signifying a worsening of their condition. Nevertheless, this is still one unit better than before they started the course of treatment, and indicates a noticeable improvement.

By comparison, the scores for the Waiting List Control Group had all remained at four during Week 6 and Week 12, the period when they received no healing. The people in this group then began their series of healing sessions from Week 13. Seven weeks after their final session, at Week 24, they completed their last set of questionnaires. At this point, they scored three for each symptom (an improvement of one point) and only two for activities (an improvement of two points).

The fact that the Waiting List Control Group followed a similar pattern of progress to that of the Intervention Group gives additional reliability to each group's results. It thereby adds further credibility to the assertion that healing has a positive effect.

The physical improvements recorded by these MYMOP scores may not have been related to symptoms of IBS or IBD. The worst problem for a patient can be something quite different. Examples of this among Dr Singh's patients include the young woman mentioned earlier who had partially lost the use of her legs; another is the woman who had suffered addictions for 30 years. After one healing session, those problems had disappeared. Had they been on the trial, their MYMOP scores would have seen massive improvement. But if they had been given questionnaires regarding IBS or IBD symptoms, their results might have been inconclusive. A similar case would be my own situation, when I had sought healing for psoriasis. The psoriasis improved a little but the main benefit was something quite different, explained later. Had I been completing a similar clutch of questionnaires to the ones used in our trial, my score for the troublesome medical condition – psoriasis – would have been mediocre, but my MYMOP score would have been excellent.

Similarly, if there were to be a detailed inspection of the completed MYMOP questionnaires in our trial, the data may reveal that a range of additional issues had been alleviated that had nothing to do with IBS or IBD. Hence, the MYMOP results are the most important of any, because the main priority of our trial was to establish whether people's lives had improved.

In the MYMOP questionnaire, one aspect of life that is measured is termed as "well-being". Despite the considerable improvements to their symptoms and quality of life, the Intervention Group did not record an equivalent enhancement to their sense of well-being, which seems odd. One would imagine that well-being should improve in line with physical improvements, but this was not reflected in the scoring.

At Week 0 they gave a more positive score – that is, three – for well-being than their distressing symptoms and impaired quality of life would suggest. They gave this same score for well-being throughout the programme, even though their symptoms had been alleviated and they were able to be more active. The Waiting List Control Group improved by one point for well-being at Week 24 (seven weeks after their final session), but the Intervention Group's deflated well-being score reduced the overall results.

Regarding the concept of "well-being", it could be that the meaning of the word is too subjective and therefore unclear to some people. Perhaps it needs to be clearly defined before asking people to give a score for it, as I had done when I conducted my hospital audits. Alternatively, the MYMOP webpage offers another explanation:

> ... treatment may change the symptoms and activity scores dramatically, and the well-being may change less because so many social and personal things affect it.

• • •

If the Intervention Group's well-being figures were not included in the total, the overall improvement figures for our trial would be greater. But even with the well-being figures included, the Intervention Group still retained significant improvements by Week 24 (p=0.002), 19 weeks after their final healing session. The phrase "p=0.002" means two in 1,000 or, simplified, odds of one in 500 against the amount of improvement occurring by chance.

As mentioned before, our researchers had specified higher significance levels than usual for our trial. For "sub-scales and domains" they had stipulated p<0.005 (less than one in 200) but for "overall" scores, they set the threshold at p<0.01 (less than one in 100). The overall MYMOP result of p=0.002 is five times better than the pre-specified level and 25 times better than the medically accepted norm of p=0.05 (one in 20).

The information presented in Figure 14 illustrates the IBS and IBD results separately, giving the overall scores for each condition including well-being. If the well-being scores were omitted, the downward trend of the curve (denoting improvement) would be even more pronounced. Nevertheless, the graph clearly shows that the two groups followed the same pattern of gains because their respective lines are virtually parallel. The lower position of the IBD line indicates that the IBD group reported less suffering than the IBS people, but the percentage of improvement was almost identical. The research paper therefore states that both groups benefited.

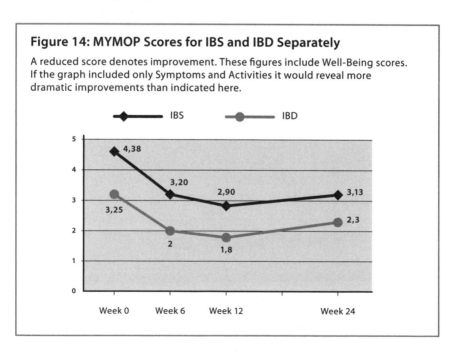

Figure 14: MYMOP Scores for IBS and IBD Separately

A reduced score denotes improvement. These figures include Well-Being scores. If the graph included only Symptoms and Activities it would reveal more dramatic improvements than indicated here.

Taking out the well-being scores shows the effect on Symptoms and Activities alone. Figure 15 – without the well-being figures – reveals a reduction of two whole points at Week 12. Comparing this with Figure 14 – which includes well-being – we see that Week 12 shows a reduction of 1.48 and 1.45 for IBS and IBD respectively (IBS 4.38-2.90=1.48 and IBD 3.25-1.80=1.45). An increase of two whole points at Week 12 is remarkable. In addition, one could easily conjecture that the level of improvement may have been greater at Week 7, 8, 9 or 10 and had begun to dissipate by Week 12.

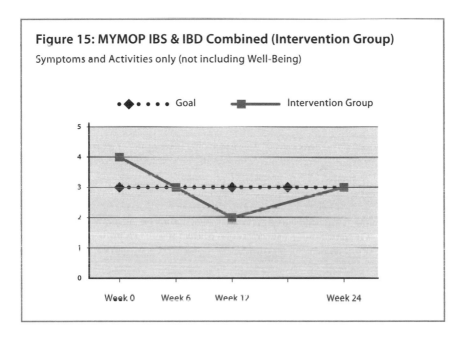

Figure 15: MYMOP IBS & IBD Combined (Intervention Group)
Symptoms and Activities only (not including Well-Being)

The quantitative research paper explains that the Waiting List Control Group generally followed the same pattern of improvement once they received their healing sessions. This was the case across all of the questionnaires. You will recall that the Waiting List Group had to wait for 12 weeks before beginning their series of healing treatments so that comparisons could be made. As an example, the MYMOP results in Figure 16 demonstrate that these patients remained static throughout the waiting period from Week 0 to Week 12. At Week 13 they began their series of five weekly healing sessions. Seven weeks later, they completed their Week 24 questionnaire where we clearly see that their improvements mirrored those of the Intervention Group. This doubly confirms the findings.

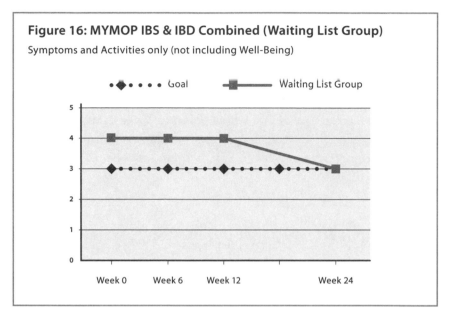

Figure 16: MYMOP IBS & IBD Combined (Waiting List Group)
Symptoms and Activities only (not including Well-Being)

These excellent MYMOP results demonstrate that the research trial achieved its primary goal. It had established that adding healing sessions to conventional treatment improves the lives of patients with IBS and also the lives of patients with IBD.

• • •

Now we turn to the specialized questionnaires that were employed to ascertain whether patients had gained improvements to quality of life issues directly relating to their particular condition.

IBS Quality of Life

In the case of people with irritable bowel syndrome (IBS), they completed the IBS-QoL questionnaire described earlier. It focuses on the particular problems that commonly affect the day-to-day lives of people with IBS. It measures the effects of the symptoms rather than the symptoms themselves.

With 34 questions, each requiring a response on a five-point scale, the score can range from 34 to 170. An increase of between ten and 14 points reflects a meaningful clinical improvement.[78] I have therefore used the midpoint of 12 for the calculation that follows.

For ease of analysis, our researchers had converted the scores to being out of 100. Mathematically, this conversion means that an increase of

12 points in the original scale – identifying clinical improvement – is equivalent to around nine points in our figures. The dotted grey line on Figure 17 on the following page is therefore at level 9 to indicate the desired goal to be achieved.

Incidentally, with the scores now being out of 100, one might presume that our results could be read as percentage improvements, but apparently not.

At Week 6, the Intervention Group (the group that received healing from the outset) gained an overall score improvement of 12.9 (p<0.001). At Week 12 the increase was 12.4 (p<0.001), and at Week 24 it was 13.8 (p<0.001). It is surprising to see a slight dip at Week 12 followed by an improvement at Week 24, which achieved a better score than Week 6.

With nine points in our figures indicating clinical improvement, the gains of 12.9, 12.4 and 13.8 must be impressive. And the "p" figures in brackets reveal that the Intervention Group improved by a statistically significant degree at each time point throughout the trial.

The improvement at Week 24 shows that benefits continued to develop after their final healing session. Gains were therefore sustained for at least 19 weeks, and could have been longer but our study was limited to a total of six months.

The Waiting List Control Group improved slightly during the 12 weeks that they waited for their healing sessions to begin. Nevertheless, even when compared to the Control Group, the Intervention Group's results remained statistically significant at Week 6 (p=0.001) and slightly less so at Week 12 (p=0.013).

Remembering that the University researchers had raised the bar for significance to p=0.01 (one in 100) for total scores, Week 6 outstripped this with p=0.001 (one in 1,000). Week 12 only just missed the elevated threshold with p=0.013 (13 in 1,000 or, simplified, 1.3 in 100).

Researchers also use "effect sizes" to convey the magnitude of improvement, and 0.8 is considered a large enough change to be noticeable.[79][80] Effect sizes give a more clinically relevant picture of health status, and are a useful tool for interpreting changes in chronic illness.[81]

The research paper explains that various adjustments were made to account for differences within the group such as age, gender and years since diagnosis.

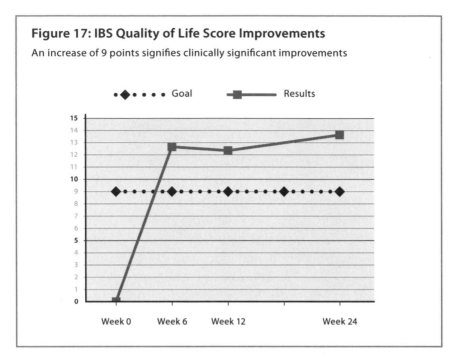

After making these adjustments, they arrived at effect sizes for the Intervention Group of 10.7 at Week 6, and 7.6 at Week 12 (see Figure 18), compared with the Control Group. I queried these seemingly outlandish figures, but they remained unchanged in the research paper so they must be correct. The dotted grey line on Figure 18 is set at 0.8 to show the level of improvement required for noticeable improvement.

An expert on the subject confirmed that 10.7 is indeed "quite extreme", but he needed more details to be able to speak directly about the impact on patients. I felt unable to provide him with further information because the research paper had not yet been published. But whether or not these figures are a cause for celebration, they remain useful for a comparison that I wish to make shortly.

Figure 18 shows the results of everyone in the group, whether or not they received all five sessions. This is referred to in the research paper as Intention To Treat (ITT).

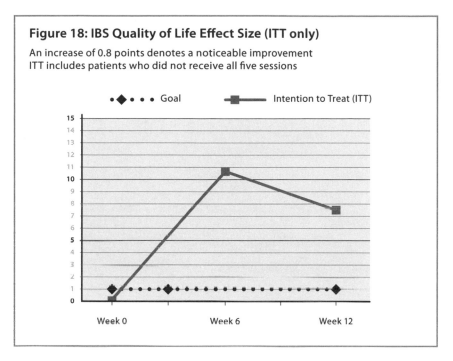

Figure 18: IBS Quality of Life Effect Size (ITT only)

An increase of 0.8 points denotes a noticeable improvement
ITT includes patients who did not receive all five sessions

The effect sizes in Figure 18 include the people who had not received all five sessions before completing their Week 6 questionnaires. As mentioned earlier, this represented 42 per cent of the Intervention Group. I should point out that 42 per cent actually refers to all of the participants as a whole, but I have assumed it would be near enough the same percentage for the IBS and IBD groups separately. If the IBS cohort had received all five of their sessions before completing the Week 6 questionnaires, there would have been better results for Week 6, Week 12 and Week 24. Let me explain how the scores substantiate this assertion.

Of the Intervention Group, 22 per cent failed to attend all five sessions. As before, 22 per cent refers to the whole Intervention Group but I have assumed the same figure for the IBS and IBD groups separately. The researchers separated out the figures for those who had received all five and found that these people had gained greater improvements than those who had fewer.

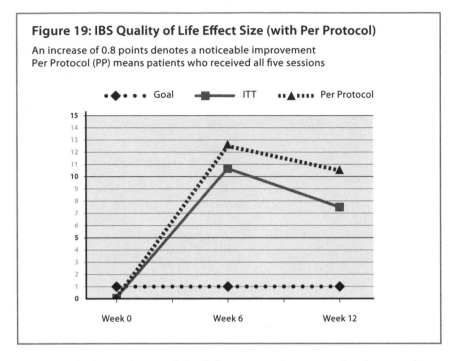

Figure 19: IBS Quality of Life Effect Size (with Per Protocol)

An increase of 0.8 points denotes a noticeable improvement
Per Protocol (PP) means patients who received all five sessions

Figure 19 helps understand the following explanation. On the same basis as the various adjustments detailed before, the effect sizes for those who received all five (per protocol) were 12.6 at Week 6, and 10.4 at Week 12, compared with the Control Group. These figures reveal that, by having attended all five sessions, they had gained an additional 1.9 effect size points at Week 6 (12.6 minus 10.7=1.9) and an additional 2.8 points at Week 12 (10.4 minus 7.6=2.8).

Thus, we can see that the score for the whole Intervention Group was dragged down by 2.8 points at Week 12 by only 22 per cent of the group – the ones who had fewer than five sessions. This means that the scores for the 22 per cent must have been substantially lower than for the 78 per cent who had all five.

These figures demonstrate that each session brings increased benefits. It therefore follows that the Week 6 figures would have been better if all participants had received their five sessions before completing the Week 6 questionnaires.

As well as this, the 78 per cent who had all five sessions retained more of the benefits by Week 12 (12.6 minus 10.4, giving a loss of 2.2 effect size points) than the Intervention Group as a whole (10.7 minus 7.6, giving a loss of 3.1 effect size points). The people who had all five sessions therefore retained an additional 0.9 effect size over the Intervention Group as a whole (3.1-2.2=0.9). If 0.8 is considered a noticeable improvement, then it must be worth retaining this additional 0.9.

Again, the above comparison is between the 78 per cent who had all five sessions and the whole (100 per cent) Intervention Group. But the whole Intervention Group includes the 78 per cent who had all five. If we compared the scores for the 78 per cent (who had all five) against only the 22 per cent (who had fewer) a greater difference would be revealed.

These calculations show that if all of the participants had received all five sessions, there would have been better results at Week 12 for IBS sufferers. And since more benefits were retained in the longer term by having all five, then the Week 24 figures would also have been enhanced.

Looking at the Intervention Group's Week 24, this was 19 weeks after their final session so one might assume that gains may have dissipated. However, the scores are better for every aspect, showing that benefits had not only been maintained but also continued to increase between Week 12 and Week 24. If everyone had received all five sessions before Week 6, there would have been a longer period for this trend to continue. Thus, the Week 24 scores could have been greater.

The majority of people had their final healing session seven weeks before Week 12 so it is intriguing to see improvements continuing to develop for so long afterwards. This positive trend could have continued beyond Week 24 but, as stated before, six months was the extent of our study.

The results of the IBS Quality of Life questionnaire (IBS-QoL) were found to be consistent with the findings of the MYMOP scores, thereby further confirming the reliability of both. With the questions being focused specifically on the issues associated with IBS, a greater insight was gained regarding the aspects of life that had improved. Almost all dimensions of quality of life within the Intervention Group exhibited at least a ten-point improvement at Week 12 and this was maintained to Week 24. Remembering that an increase of about nine points in our figures (by the reckoning explained earlier) conveys clinical significance, these are excellent results. Mood, outlook, activities, food issues, attitude, social life and sex life had all achieved a level of improvement that was noticeable to the patient.

The results of this questionnaire further confirmed that the research trial had achieved one of its primary goals. It had established that healing sessions improve quality of life issues that particularly affect patients with IBS.

IBD Quality of Life

Turning now to the people in the inflammatory bowel disease (IBD) group, they completed the IBDQ questionnaire described previously. It was designed specifically to measure the quality of life experienced by people with this particular condition. As opposed to the IBS-QoL, which does not ask about physical symptoms, the IBDQ devotes three-fifths of its questions to bowel problems and to general physical health.

Despite the difference in focus, the IBDQ results followed a similar pattern to the IBS-QoL, with the Intervention Group demonstrating a significant overall improvement at Week 6 (p=0.008) and even more so at Week 12 (p<0.001).

The questionnaire consists of 32 questions that are scored by the patient on a seven-point scale, giving a range of possible scores from 32 to 224. Higher scores indicate a better quality of life, an improvement of 20 points denoting clinical significance.[82]

As with the IBS-QoL, our researchers had converted the actual IBDQ scores into being out of 100 for easier analysis. Mathematically, this must mean that an increase of about ten points in our trial's figures denotes a clinically significant improvement. The dotted grey line on Figure 20 is therefore at level 10 to indicate the level of improvement required for noticeable improvement. The dotted grey line on Figure 20 is therefore at level 10 to indicate the level of improvement required for noticeable improvement.

The two main problems regarding bowel function improved by 11.6 points (p=0.006) and 14.2 points (p=0.022) respectively by Week 12.

This shows that symptom improvements were retained and even increased over the seven weeks following their final healing session. There was a reduction over the following three months but they were still better off at Week 24 (p=0.044) than before joining the trial.

Again, we see that score improvements were greater at Week 12 than they had been at Week 6. The two dimensions that gained the most improvement were "bowel function" (p <0.001) and "social function" (p<0.001) at Week 12. Naturally, if a person's bowels are more predictable and less painful, social situations can be engaged in with more confidence and enjoyment.

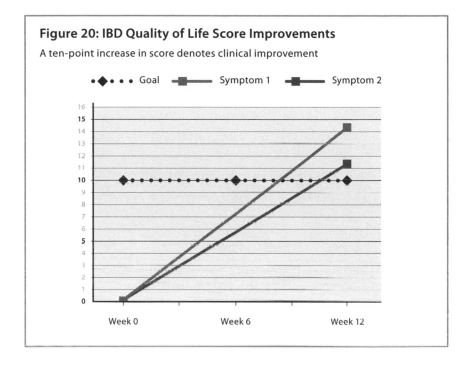

Figure 20: IBD Quality of Life Score Improvements

A ten-point increase in score denotes clinical improvement

Goal · · · · · Symptom 1 ▬■▬ Symptom 2 ▬■▬

After making the various adjustments referred to earlier regarding age etc., the Intervention Group achieved effect sizes of 5.8 at Week 6 and 10.1 at Week 12 (p=0.004) compared with the Control Group. Again, these seem surprisingly high figures if 0.8 is considered noticeable to a patient.

When the researchers separated out the results for people who had received all five sessions, they found that the scores were almost the same whether people had the full quota or less. There had been a notable difference between these figures for the IBS patients (IBS-QoL). But the IBD questionnaire had a stronger focus on physical symptoms, which could be an explanation. The researchers also thought the disparity may be due to IBS and IBD being different medical conditions.

The Week 24 figure for the Intervention Group could be expected to be worse than any other figure because this would be 19 weeks after their final session. Indeed, the figures are all slightly worse but most of the improvements had been retained. Again, these benefits may have lasted longer but our study was limited to a total of six months.

Overall, the researchers found that the IBDQ results were consistent with the findings of the MYMOP scores, which further confirms the reliability of both.

The results of this questionnaire again verified that the research trial had achieved one of its primary goals. It had established that adding healing sessions to conventional care improves the lives of patients with IBD. On their own, these excellent quality-of-life enhancements for both IBS and IBD patients, reiterated across the three different questionnaires, would be highly meaningful for the patients involved. But the secondary aim of the trial was to ascertain whether the physical symptoms characteristic of IBS and of IBD had actually been alleviated. To measure changes in the severity of symptoms, each group completed a questionnaire designed for their particular diagnosis.

IBS Symptoms

The IBS group completed the Birmingham IBS questionnaire, described earlier. Its 11 questions are scored on a six-point scale, resulting in a minimum possible score of 11 and a maximum of 66.

Results revealed that the Intervention Group's physical symptoms had gained significant improvements especially at Week 6 ($p<0.001$) compared with the Control Group. The gains were slightly reduced at Week 12 ($p=0.018$) but the research paper nevertheless confirms that the retained improvements are likely to reflect a clinically determinable effect.

The scores were slightly lower at Week 24 but, even so, were still a substantial improvement over baseline in comparison to the Control Group. In other words, patients gained significant physical improvements during the period of time that they received healing and, despite the slight decline afterwards, were better off at Week 24 than before joining the programme. Positive effects of healing had therefore been retained for 19 weeks after their final healing session and could have lasted longer.

Now the researchers could see that the results of the Birmingham IBS questionnaire were consistent with the other two that had been completed by the IBS cohort (MYMOP and IBS-QoL), further confirming that the results across all three were reliable.

From these results, it was clear that a secondary aim of the trial had been achieved. Adding healing sessions to conventional treatment had alleviated the physical symptoms of IBS patients.

IBD Symptoms

Turning now to the inflammatory bowel disease (IBD) group, this was originally intended to only include patients with ulcerative colitis. Finding enough people with this condition proved more difficult than expected, so the Steering Group had been prompted to include Crohn's disease. Crohn's is an IBD that is very similar to colitis but, in research terms, "similar" is not "the same". With the IBD group split between these two different conditions, the results cannot be compared like for like within the group as a whole. Also, the number of people within each subgroup was too small to provide meaningful analysis for either condition, or for conclusions to be drawn. Nevertheless, the results make interesting reading and are presented here.

Ulcerative Colitis Symptoms

The ulcerative colitis group used the SCCAI questionnaire described earlier to measure changes in their physical symptoms. Total scores range from 0 to 19, with a decrease denoting improvement and a score of 2.5 correlating with remission.[83] The dotted grey line on Figure 21 is therefore at level 2.5.

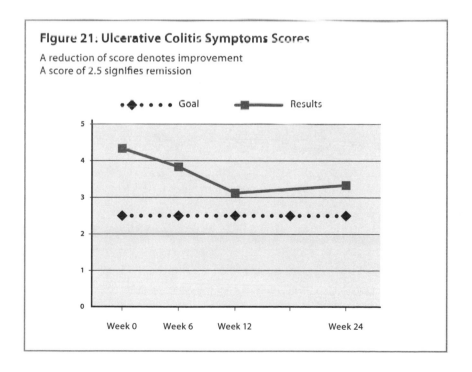

Figure 21: Ulcerative Colitis Symptoms Scores

A reduction of score denotes improvement
A score of 2.5 signifies remission

The scores for the Intervention Group reveal an improvement from 4.3 at Week 0 to 3.8 at Week 6 (p=0.41). This was followed by a further gain at Week 12 with a score of 3.1 (p=0.046). There was a small slide back up to 3.4 by Week 24 but symptoms were still better at this point than before having healing. The Waiting List Control Group followed a similar pattern, after receiving healing.

Crohn's Disease Symptoms

To establish whether symptoms improved for the Crohn's disease group, these patients used the H-B questionnaire described before. Again, a reduction of score signifies an improvement in symptoms, with 13 denoting extreme severity. A score of less than five is considered to represent clinical remission.[84] The dotted grey line on Figure 22 is therefore at level 5.

The Intervention Group's score began at 8.5 at Week 0, reducing to 7.9 at Week 6, and down again to 7.0 by Week 12. At Week 24 it was down to a remarkable 4.4, a score indicating clinical remission.

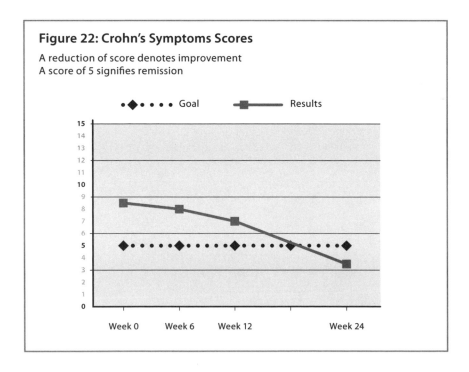

Figure 22: Crohn's Symptoms Scores
A reduction of score denotes improvement
A score of 5 signifies remission

This signifies that outstanding improvements continued to develop between seven and 19 weeks after their final healing session. The natural question that arises is: How could the improvements during this latter period be due to the placebo effect if these patients were not receiving the care and attention that is deemed to activate it? The Waiting List Control Group set off with a Week 0 score of 6.7. They then waited for 12 weeks before beginning their healing sessions. Their Week 12 figure showed that nothing had particularly changed for them since Week 0. They then began to receive their series of healing sessions. Seven weeks later, at Week 24, their score had reduced to 4.3. They had improved by the same surprising degree as the Intervention Group, but more quickly.

These are astounding results, but the Crohn's group consisted of only 24 people. In research terms, this is too small a sample size to be statistically convincing. Consequently, although these scores appear in the table presented in the research paper, they are not mentioned within the text. But since both the Intervention Group and the Waiting List Control Group improved by the same extraordinary degree, then surely further investigation is warranted. Added to this, the Intervention Group revealed increasing benefits for 19 weeks after their final session – and this trend could have lasted longer. The Waiting List Control Group may have fared equally well in the longer term, but this was well beyond the extent of our study.

Again, from the results of these two different IBD questionnaires, a secondary aim of the trial had been achieved. It had established that receiving healing sessions had alleviated the physical symptoms of IBD, though not convincingly in academic research terms.

A similar study with larger numbers in each IBD group would, of course, be more persuasive for scientists, but ulcerative colitis and Crohn's are not common diseases. Considering that a sufficient number of patients with ulcerative colitis could not be found for our trial in Birmingham – Britain's second biggest city – the results of our study may have to suffice for the time being. Clearly, a study of Crohn's disease would be even more challenging to populate.

Overall

There were 105 IBS patients in our study, a sufficient number from which to gain reliable statistical results in relation to IBS. The IBD group as a whole was also sizeable with 94 patients but it had to be split between 70 colitis and 24 Crohn's patients. The smaller the group is, the less dependable the statistical data analysis becomes. For the

Crohn's group in particular, no conclusions have been drawn within the research paper.

Each of the three questionnaires completed by participants supported the findings of the other two. The questions were different in each one so the results naturally varied, but there remained substantial consistency across them all. For example, the MYMOP scores for the IBS people were compatible with the results of their IBS-QoL and Birmingham IBS questionnaires, and the same can be seen across the IBD cohort. This compatibility lends additional credibility to the findings of each one.

The researchers noted the difference in symptom benefits between the IBS and IBD groups and suggested that this could be because they are unrelated conditions, as outlined earlier.

With the IBS symptom improvements being more pronounced and lasting longer, the researchers suggest that people with functional disorders might be more disposed to benefiting from healing sessions than people with actual physical disease. The term "functional disorder" refers to any medical condition that impairs the normal function of a bodily process, but where every part of the body looks completely normal under examination, dissection or under a microscope. Irritable bowel syndrome is not a disease, and there is no physical cause for the symptoms to occur, yet they are known to be exacerbated by emotional upset and stress.

Inflammatory bowel disease, on the other hand, does have physical causes for the symptoms to occur, though nobody knows what triggers the disease into existence in the first place.

But physical symptoms were the secondary focus of our investigation. Improving lives was the primary concern, and the MYMOP results confirm that this was achieved equally for both IBS and IBD patients.

In summation, from the quantitative data in front of them, the researchers were able to draw conclusions. Considering the controversial nature of the study, we could expect their statements to be cautious and fully considered. Each of the authors would no doubt wish to protect their professional and academic reputation. In addition, the University of Birmingham's executive is likely to have ensured that its internal peer review process was particularly rigorous.

The following statements appear in the research paper. First of all, regarding all participants, they confirmed that healing makes a positive difference:

*Results demonstrate that when used alongside standard medical
care, healing therapy confers additional benefit.*

They pointed out that the patients who received all five sessions – referred
to as "per protocol" – benefited more than those who received fewer. This
confirms that each additional session brought increased benefits:

*Per protocol analyses suggested that greater benefit was associated
with compliance, further supporting the observed findings.*

In respect of the MYMOP scores measuring quality of life for all participants, whether they had IBS or IBD, they stated that:

*Changes in scores were of a size with the potential to result in notable
improvements to the patient.*

*We have observed that healing therapy is beneficial, both in terms of
improvement in patient perception of disease impact (determined by
MYMOP), which was our pre-specified primary outcome.*

In respect of the MYMOP results for the Intervention Group, which
included both IBS and IBD, the research paper confirms that benefits
remained for many weeks after their final healing sessions and could have
lasted longer:

*... all symptom and activity measures (except for well-being) showed
improvements which were maintained up to Week 24, suggesting the
possibility of longer-term benefits beyond the period of therapy.*

In respect of IBS patients, they confirmed the substantial benefits gained:

*Benefits observed in our IBS cohort in terms of both symptom
reduction and quality of life improvement were significant, consistent
and of size likely to be associated with clinical benefit.*

The term "clinical benefit" refers to noticeable improvements that are
important to the patient. A further statement reminds us that these
patients had continued to be ill despite a range of orthodox treatment
administered over a prolonged period of time:

*This study has demonstrated that clinically there is benefit to be
gained from inclusion of healing in the management of IBS that has
not responded to conventional management.*

Of course, it would be more useful to provide healing at a much earlier stage. Why wait until all conventional treatments have been tried? Regarding the IBS group, the researchers confirmed that significant benefits had been gained, which had lasted for many weeks after their final healing session:

> Quality of life was considerably enhanced in the IBS Intervention Group with improvements in emotional states, socialization, and activity levels which were maintained up to Week 24 and were significantly different from controls.

Continuing to talk about the IBS results, the research paper states that the Waiting List Control Group improved similarly once they had received their series of healing sessions, and that this was commensurate with the MYMOP results:

> Parallel to observations made in the MYMOP data, there was a meaningful improvement in the quality of life scores for the Control Group once they also received the intervention.

The researchers reached the conclusion that adding healing to conventional care increases benefits to IBS and IBD patients:

> The addition of healing therapy to conventional treatment was associated with improvement in symptoms and quality of life in IBS, and to a lesser extent in IBD.

> This pragmatic trial demonstrates that patient benefit is accrued through the addition of healing therapy to conventional management of both IBS and IBD.

A pragmatic trial is a randomized controlled trial that evaluates the effectiveness of an intervention in real-life, routine practice conditions.[85]

In addition, the researchers suggested that other conditions could benefit from healing:

> These findings may suggest that conditions linked to functional disorders could accrue greater benefit from healing therapy.

Other functional disorders include fibromyalgia, chronic fatigue syndrome, migraine and tension headaches, chronic pelvic pain, interstitial cystitis and other conditions.[86]

The placebo effect is invariably pointed to when a medical benefit has been gained without drugs or surgery. However, in our study, the effects were considered too great to be attributable to placebo alone:

The benefit observed may at least be, in part, a placebo effect although the size of benefits observed suggests an alternative mechanism.

In any case, the researchers advised that the benefit to patients should be the main concern, not whether the method can be understood:

The value of any mechanism should not be discounted where it confers symptomatic relief.

These are all particularly powerful statements, especially when set against the backdrop of extreme prudence described earlier. In addition, they confirmed that these findings are in keeping with previous research:

Results from this study are analogous to the conclusions made by ... previous studies which generally support the effectiveness of healing therapy to reduce pain, anxiety and improved quality of life.

They also made the observation that healing is safe and a positive experience for recipients:

We found no evidence of harm from healing therapy.

Many patients found it to be an interesting and enjoyable experience.

They positively recommended that healing be administered to patients:

Patients with IBS and IBD seen in secondary care, who remain symptomatic despite the best medical care, should be considered for healing therapy, where this is available, with the understanding that benefit is likely to be greater in individuals with IBS.

This statement points to potentially greater benefit for IBS symptoms than IBD. But the IBD group did gain benefits, and most especially the Crohn's sufferers. However, symptoms were a secondary focus of our research programme. The main concern was whether lives had improved, and this was confirmed by the MYMOP results, which showed that the IBS and IBD groups gained equally.

Almost all of these patients were receiving specialist medical attention immediately prior to joining the programme. Naturally, they would have already benefited from any placebo effect that is deemed to be triggered by professional care and attention. They had exhausted all of the treatments offered by their GP and were now at varying stages of receiving specialist care. The minimum time that any of these patients had suffered was 18 months since diagnosis. Many had been receiving specialist treatment for years, one of them for over a decade.

It is worth reiterating that, since healing has been found to be effective, it would make sense to administer this therapy long before the patient reaches the stage of needing a consultant.

It was fantastic to have scientific confirmation from a top-ranking university, known for high-quality research, that our healing work was markedly beneficial to patients. Of course, the researchers made it clear that they did not know by which mechanism the benefits had occurred. The study was designed solely to establish whether healing sessions made a difference to people affected by chronic IBS or IBD. This was confirmed, and convincingly so.

Observations

The various questionnaires used in this trial scored in opposite ways to each other. Improvements were conveyed by an increase in score for some and by a decrease in others. It would be less confusing if there were a standardized method of presenting results. It would be seem appropriate to designate 0 as "no symptoms", with increasing scores linked to escalating severity.

It was very difficult to track down the text of research papers that I wanted to reference throughout the book. Had I been affiliated to an academic or medical institution, I would have had the luxury of unlimited access. But as I am an ordinary member of the public, it took a great deal of time and effort to locate even the simplest information. One example was trying to find out how many points of increase or decrease in score constitutes clinical significance in respect of each of the questionnaires. One would think that the public should be able to access medical research information if they wanted to but, in the main, it is not possible without paying multiple and expensive subscriptions.

The data for our trial were collected specifically to answer the research questions that were posed at the outset. But additional research is possible using the same raw data. Usually, the same researchers will develop a new research question that the existing data can answer. This is a time-efficient and cost-effective method of gaining further insights, and can lead to a number of research papers being published. Researchers from any other organization ought to be allowed access to the data for our trial because it was funded by public money via the Lottery. It seems obvious that the next step would be to ascertain, using the same data, whether particular elements within the protocol helped to maximize or prolong the beneficial effects of receiving healing sessions.

For instance, a closer inspection might reveal whether patients who saw the same healer for all five sessions benefited more than those who saw multiple healers. Typically, each new patient is so impressed with their first healing session that they want to continue with the same healer. But when they do have to see someone else, they are almost always pleasantly surprised. Although patients might initially feel disconcerted, it would be useful to know if the healing outcome is affected. On our trial, all appointments for each participant were intended to be with the same healer, but it was not always possible. Consequently, there should be enough patients in each category to identify a difference.

Also, we know from the research paper that people gained more if they received all five sessions. In addition, I have explained how the scores reveal the degree to which these people benefited more, including in the longer term. But another potentially valuable point would be to know if the people who received all five healing sessions within five weeks gained better results than those whose appointments were spread over a longer period.

And did the people who had five in five weeks also benefit more in the longer term, as would be identified by their Week 24 figures? We know that 42 per cent of participants had not received all five sessions when they completed their Week 6 questionnaire so there will be enough people in each category to make a comparison.

It would be useful to know whether the people with the worst symptoms gained the most improvements, as reported in other healing trials. A closer inspection of the data might show whether this was equally the case for IBS and IBD. If so, the obvious course of action would be to offer a series of regular healing sessions to all people suffering severe IBS or IBD symptoms.

And did patients benefit more if they were invited to join the programme by a consultant who imparted some confidence in the therapy? Dr Singh was in a position to convey, from first-hand knowledge, that many patients had been helped by healing sessions and that they had found it enjoyable. Other consultants, however – especially those external to Dr Singh's clinic – are unlikely to have been so encouraging, and this may have affected the outcome. Again, there should be enough patients in each category to make a comparison. If there were a difference between the two groups, this would highlight the value of a supportive recommendation given by a consultant, and would identify an element of the placebo effect in action. If there were no difference, this would be in keeping with my own observations where patients benefited despite their consultant's scepticism. If a future trial were to be conducted, additional questions could be incorporated to investigate this aspect. The patient could be asked to give a score for how confident and assuring the consultant seemed when offering healing, and also a score for how beneficial they themselves thought that healing might be.

An examination of the raw data might also reveal how many participants made an instant and full recovery, like the teenager described in an earlier chapter (page 92). One person did quit the programme after their first session, saying that all of the symptoms had disappeared. As she had been suffering from the condition for quite some time, this was an excellent outcome. However, because the patient did not continue, this data could not be included in the study figures. There may have been others who quit for the same reason. Obviously, our research results would have been even better if these people had continued in the programme.

Patients who have a swift and full recovery may have certain traits or attitudes in common. A future trial could aim to identify these so that others have the opportunity to emulate them. Equally, it would be interesting to know whether anyone who attended all five sessions felt they had gained nothing. However, very few people could have fallen into these two extreme categories, because the results are expressed with 95 per cent certainty that an identical trial would produce similar findings.

I mentioned earlier that the Intervention Group's Week 0 to Week 12 improvements could be expected to be similar to the Waiting List Control Group's Week 12 to Week 24 results. As mentioned before,

Figure 13 (page 129) makes it easier to understand that these two periods for the respective groups are equivalent to each other. The only difference between the two is that the Waiting List Group had waited for 12 weeks before beginning their sessions. The Waiting List Control Group generally gained slightly less than the Intervention Group in respect of physical symptoms. If this is actually the case, patients would clearly benefit more if they embarked on healing sessions right away, rather than having to wait for any length of time.

Regarding Week 12 and Week 24 figures, some of the results suggest that certain positive effects dissipated over time. However, a different explanation for lower scores could be provided by a well-known concept within social science that says, in essence, that today's perceptions become tomorrow's expectations.[87] When people repeatedly experience a higher level of quality, this becomes the norm for them, and what used to be acceptable is now considered substandard.

In the context of our trial, a patient gives a particular score for their current health and a higher score later on if they improve; but if the improvement remains for several weeks, this new level of health becomes their normal expectation – it no longer has the "wow" factor that it once had. As a result, the patient is likely to give this heightened level of health a lower score than they would have before, even though it is actually the same. Thus, the Week 12 and especially the Week 24 scores could have been marked lower than would reflect the actual health of the patient. If this is the case, then the positive effects may not have dissipated over time, even if the figures might suggest so in some of the results. Also, this would mean that the scores that did improve at Week 24 are particularly striking.

As explained, all clinical research results include comparisons between the control group (the group that had no treatment) and the group that did receive the treatment. The people in the control group often improve slightly despite having had no treatment or attention, and this occurred in some aspects of our trial. Accordingly, the benefits gained by our participants would be even more impressive if compared to patients who did not take part in the programme. And the difference must be greater than our study indicates.

By the time our trial participants completed their Week 0 questionnaires, at least a few weeks had elapsed since they were originally invited to take part. The Hawthorne findings, described on page 67, would suggest that the placebo effect should spring into action at the point of being asked to be part of a trial – the time at which they first received attention – not a few weeks later, after completing the Week 0 paperwork. If so, our Week 0 figures will actually be better than if the forms had been completed at the time these patients were first approached.

It follows that the Week 0 figures will also be better than for patients who did not take part at all. The real difference, then, between those who received healing and those who did not take part in the programme, will be greater than shown in our figures.

It would be intriguing to know if there is an even greater disparity in respect of the people who flatly refused to take part on the basis that they thought that spiritual healing would be a waste of time. To find out, a future study could ask these patients to simply complete the same questionnaires as the trial participants. If doing this contravenes RCT protocols, perhaps it is time to review the rules.

• • •

Our research results confirmed that healing sessions are beneficial to patients. A future trial could aim to ascertain whether these positive effects could be maximized and/or prolonged by adjusting the protocol. The following ideas could provide a starting point. People who received all five healing sessions gained greater improvements than those who had fewer. The next step would be to discover whether additional sessions bring about ever-increasing benefits, and, if so, how many.

The Week 24 figures confirm that benefits were maintained over the longer term, but it would be useful to know how long they continued beyond this point. Although an extended trial would take a long time to gain the answer, the process would give more patients the opportunity to benefit from healing sessions while waiting to find out.

In addition, it would be worth investigating whether it is possible to actively prolong the beneficial effects. Perhaps ongoing monthly sessions would provide an effective maintenance level.

Qualitative Results

To gain a more comprehensive appreciation of how healing had affected actual lives, qualitative explanatory data was gained by interviewing 22 of the participants.[88]

In research terms, these interviews add what is called triangulation. This means that more than one method has been used to check the results. It gives more confidence in the results when different methods lead to the same findings. Triangulation has been defined as:

> ... an attempt to map out, or explain more fully, the richness and complexity of human behaviour by studying it from more than one standpoint.[89]

To improve the uniformity of the interviewing process the participants were selected by one of the University researchers, and they were all interviewed by him. With only one researcher involved in this element of the study, the one-to-one sessions were more likely to be conducted in a consistent manner. Of the 22 people he interviewed, 13 had IBS, six had ulcerative colitis and three had Crohn's disease.

These interviews took place at the hospital immediately after their final healing session. The results of a healing session are not necessarily evident directly afterwards, so there may well have been more benefits to report if the interviews had been a few days later. However, it was more convenient for people to be seen while they were already at the hospital, rather than asking them to make an additional trip.

The University researcher first asked if they had known of healing in any way before they were introduced to the programme. Of the 22 people interviewed:

- Six had no prior knowledge of healing.
- Two had friends who had benefited from healing.
- Four had received some form of healing in the past.

• • •

I was surprised that as many as four people out of the 22 had received healing before. Barely any of the 267 people included in my hospital audits said that they had experienced healing before, when asked. Perhaps one explanation could be that some of the patients included in the trial had, at an earlier time, received healing at the hospital after an appointment with Dr Singh.

Reading all of the interview comments, there is not one patient who said they believed that healing could help. Moreover, their statements underlined their prior scepticism. Nevertheless, they stated that they had entered into the sessions with an open mind and were curious as to what might happen. During the interviews, it transpired that:

- Nine felt that they had benefited physically.
- Eleven reported benefiting in other ways.
- Ten said the sessions made them feel more relaxed or calm.
- Six were not aware of any improvements or were unsure.

Regarding physical sensations while receiving healing, they reported the following impressions:

- Seven felt localized warmth or heat.
- Three identified a sense of energy.
- Three felt involuntary muscle jumps.
- Two reported feeling uplifted.
- Two saw bright colours or light.
- One had visions.

The interviewer then asked about their experience in more detail and found that the majority of their responses were in keeping with each other. Their verbatim statements are publicly available online within the research paper. For brevity, I have paraphrased them, but the unabridged text gives a richer picture. A number of the comments that follow were made by more than one patient.

First, the interviewer asked how they had felt during the sessions. They described an especially positive relationship with their respective healer that was based on trust and confidence.

- The healer looks after you.
- The healer is marvellous.
- The healer seems to relax you immediately.
- The healer has empathy with you.
- The way the healer speaks is calming.
- Extremely relaxing.
- Your whole body sinks.
- All the tension left.
- I have learned how to relax.

- Felt like "me" time.
- Felt nurturing.
- Every session was a different experience.

He then asked for more details about any physical sensations experienced during the healing session.

- Intense heat.
- Heat from the healer's hands.
- The healer's hands were cold yet felt heat in the body where the hands were.
- Temperature of healer's hands alternated between hot and cold.
- As though a bright light in the room.
- Tingling.
- Involuntary muscle spasms.
- Sensation of being pulled.
- Pain gone.
- Felt heat where pain was. Now feels better.

All of the above observations are commonly reported by patients and serve to demonstrate that more must be happening than meets the eye. They are sensations that do not normally happen when simply relaxing.

The interviewer asked these patients whether the healing sessions had made an ongoing difference to their lives. They mainly remarked upon how calm they generally felt, and that they were now far less likely to worry than before.

- Can now get on with life.
- Much calmer now.
- Take things in my stride now.
- No longer get worked up.
- No longer tense.
- Can relax now.
- Less likely to agonize over things now.
- Can switch off now.
- Calm now, despite life's difficulties.
- Can stop myself stressing now.

Regarding the difference to their physical symptoms, patients reported a range of improvements. The people who found that they had less dependency on bathrooms now enjoyed the freedom to go out and lead a more normal life. Any improvement of their symptoms must have been an enormous help to them.

- Have not needed to take sick leave from work.
- Sick less.
- Less stomach cramping.
- Less diarrhoea.
- Less pain.
- Able to be more active.
- Bowels more normal.
- Taking less medication.
- No longer choking.
- Less bloating.
- Visiting the toilet less often.
- Managed a full shift at work.
- Didn't need the bathroom all day.
- Swelling seems reduced.
- Spring in my step now.
- Feeling happier.
- Feel full of life after a healing session.

As seen in my two hospital audits, another commonly reported phenomenon regarding the effects of healing is that people often sleep better. Good-quality sleep is a healer in itself, and patients said that they had noticed the following:

- Sleeping better.
- Sleeping is a big benefit.
- More satisfying sleep.
- Sleep brilliantly after a healing session.
- Sleeping very well now.

Patients also reported coping better with their symptoms and generally had a more positive mental attitude.

A better frame of mind is a great advantage and helps people to feel more in control, more confident and happier.

- Improved perception.
- Feeling positive about the illness now.
- Positive outlook transfers to people around me.
- Dealing with things better.
- Now changing my thinking patterns for the better.
- More clear-headed.
- More open to situations now.
- Feel able to do things for myself now.
- Leading a more independent life now.
- Happier because no longer dependent upon toilets.
- Starting to get back on track.
- Symptoms no longer depress me.
- Handling situations in a more positive way.
- Able to deal with things in a more relaxed way.
- Feeling more confident.
- No longer letting the illness control me.
- Getting back to how I was before the illness.
- Feeling cleansed.
- More alert.
- No longer feeling angry about being ill.
- No longer take additional pills during a flare-up.
- No longer excessively worried about access to toilets.

• • •

In their totality, the above responses to the respective questions reiterate that healing can help physically, mentally and emotionally. Considering how long these people had suffered for, they must have thoroughly appreciated the improvements they noticed. And so must their loved ones.

Observations

In addition to the significantly positive results, the research paper refers to the many patients who stated that they found the experience to be interesting and enjoyable. At one of the final Steering Group meetings, the University researchers commented that they themselves had enjoyed being involved in this particular trial. They also remarked on the especially high take-up by patients invited to enrol, and the very low drop-out rate during the programme. The healers were delighted to be involved and the patients clearly benefited, so it is true to say that this was a particularly successful clinical trial in all respects.

It is reassuring to note the similarities between what these patients told the researcher during their interviews and the comments made by my 267 audit patients. When speaking to me, it would be natural for people to be polite and positive about a session that I had just given them, and perhaps even more so if they knew that I was a volunteer. However, the wish to please the healer is removed if the patient is speaking to a third party, in this case the researcher. It was satisfying to see that the range of positive responses given to him echoed those provided to me by the audit patients. The results of our research trial had therefore further confirmed the validity of my two hospital audits.

I was taken aback to discover that one of the interviewed patients had found healing to be painful and highly emotional during and after every session. I had never heard of this happening to anyone before. However, despite what sounded like an ordeal, this person nevertheless maintained a very positive relationship with the healer, attended all five appointments and felt confident that every session had been highly beneficial.

Each time I greeted a patient on the research trial whom I had seen the week before, I would ask how they had fared in the meantime. Not one of them told me of an adverse reaction or of any concerns that they had about their experience. Only tiredness afterwards was mentioned, and this is often the case. Many healers believe that feeling tired is the body's way of encouraging the patient to rest so that it can focus all available energy on healing itself. When people allow themselves to respond to this weariness by having a nap, they usually notice how very much better they feel afterwards. One of Dr Singh's patients told me that she was so extremely tired after a healing session that her husband thought she had been drugged. But after an unusually long and deep sleep she felt renewed and full of vim, and this improvement endured.

By employing multiple healers, the positive results of this research trial demonstrate that a patient does not need to be dependent upon one particular healer. I was the only healer involved in my two hospital audits, and the impressive results might give people the notion that I am a particularly gifted healer. But the research trial employed three main healers plus a few others when needed and the patients nevertheless improved in very similar ways. Countless healers speak of comparable outcomes for their patients and, as we used a variety of healers, our research trial shows that their claims could well be true.

Since all the healers employed on the trial were members of the Healing Trust, the results indicate that any patient could expect to benefit in similar ways by using healers trained in the same method. My own opinion is that the precise system of healing is not so important. So long as the healer has been trained properly, I believe that it is the amount of passion behind the intent to heal that really matters.

The Placebo Effect

Whatever the results of our healing trial, scientists and doctors are likely to point to the placebo effect as being the only cause of any improvements. It is therefore worth taking a closer look at this remarkable phenomenon.

The word "placebo" is Latin for "I shall please" and conveys that the pill or treatment given will do nothing more than please the patient. It may be tempting, then, to think that the placebo effect is simply the patient's innate self-healing in action. It is, in part — but this cannot be the whole story. Placebo can only apply to humans who have faith in a treatment. It clearly cannot apply to plants or animals, or human tissue in Petri dishes. Abundant research gives clear evidence that something other than placebo must be causing the improvements in these non-human subjects. The placebo effect is generated from within the patient themselves, whereas the healing seen in non-human subjects can only have been stimulated by an external energy source. Patients who receive healing must benefit from both, and our results support this suggestion.

Scientists and the medical fraternity may contend that the placebo effect is the only means by which our patients improved. This would be the same as saying that healers have learned how to harness the power of the placebo effect over and above the level that best medical care and attention can achieve. If that is the case, surely all medical professionals should learn to do likewise and/or employ healers to provide this valuable aspect of healthcare.

As we have discussed, our trial was not able to include a placebo. Instead it simply focused on whether the health and well-being of IBS and IBD patients could be further improved by having healing sessions.

Looking back to my audit graphs, we can see the improvements gained by patients immediately after their consultation with Dr Singh. In each category, the grey columns all nudged towards the "Excellent" end, suggesting that the placebo effect had been activated. We can assume, then, that these patients achieved the maximum placebo gains that could be hoped for by receiving best medical attention.

The towering white columns at the "Excellent" ends after they had their healing sessions reveal dramatic improvements in every graph. Can it be reasonable to say that this level of further benefit is attributable only to placebo?

Scientists have sought to understand the placebo effect for many years, with mixed findings.

In 1955, Henry Beecher, a Boston medical doctor, published his classic work *The Powerful Placebo*.[90] Based on the results of over 1,000 patients, he calculated that around 35 per cent of people gain a high degree of benefit from the use of a placebo.

However, in 1997, two German scientists reviewed 800 articles and stated that Beecher's work was no more than fiction.[91]

Soon afterwards, two medical doctors at the National Hospital of Denmark conducted a systematic review and concluded that placebos had no significant effects for physically measurable outcomes, and only small benefits for subjective outcomes such as well-being and pain.[92]

More in line with Beecher, Professor Fabrizio Benedetti at the University of Turin demonstrated that placebos reduce the firing of neurons, thereby enabling Parkinson's disease patients to move more easily. Also supporting Beecher's findings, Harvard Medical School conducted a study in 2008 that leaves little doubt that the placebo effect is real and powerful.[93] However, their protocol attracted participants who most likely believed in the therapy employed. This and other factors geared the trial to maximizing the placebo effect and their highly positive findings have been the most referenced in subsequent articles.

Professor Ted Kaptchuk, one of the researchers involved in the Harvard study, says that placebo treatments have been found to stimulate physical responses such as heart rate, blood pressure, chemical activity in the brain, pain, depression, anxiety, fatigue and some symptoms of Parkinson's disease. He believes that we should be working to maximize the placebo effect. To dismiss the placebo effect, he says, ignores a huge chunk of healthcare that caregivers could be utilizing.

In his book *The Placebo Effect in Alternative Medicine: Can the Performance of a Healing Ritual Have Clinical Significance?*, Kaptchuk discusses alternative therapies that produce a more positive outcome than a proven, specific, conventional treatment. For these cases, he questions why a conventional treatment should be thought more legitimate than an alternative therapy.

An extraordinary example of the power of placebo was demonstrated by an RCT of 165 patients. Medical staff simulated knee operations, cutting and sewing up the skin to give a convincing scar, and following up with the usual aftercare. Assessments over a two-year period showed that there was no difference between the groups at any point. Pain relief and their ability to walk and climb stairs had improved whether they had received the real operation or the fake one.[94] A subsequent study of 145 patients produced similar results.[95]

Studies on placebo at the University of Colorado have shown that activity drops in the brain areas that process pain, and increases in areas involved in emotion. Rather than blocking pain signals, it seems that the placebo may be changing how the brain interprets pain.[96] And this trait is thought to be passed on in our genes.[97] If positive emotion cuts off pain this may be why so many people in my two audits reported relief from pain coupled with a heightened sense of well-being. One would naturally expect to feel happier at the reduction or elimination of pain. But the Colorado research turns that sequence on its head and shows that upliftment occurs first, *then* pain reduction.

Other research shows that there is no particular type of person who is more susceptible to placebos. Age, gender, intelligence, personality traits and religious beliefs have no relevance.[98] In addition, a person who responds to a placebo on one occasion may not do so on the next.

The following five disparate groups of people have been shown to report similar experiences after receiving healing:

1. People who actively sought healing by visiting a healing centre, and were therefore likely to be optimistic regarding its efficacy.
2. People who were offered the opportunity to try healing when attending their support groups, such as MND or breast cancer. They did not seek healing but were likely to think they had nothing to lose.
3. Medical professionals who did not seek healing but accepted the opportunity while attending the Nursing in Practice exhibitions. Some were open-minded; most were sceptical.
4. The 267 hospital patients included in my two audits. They had no prior intention of having healing, and most were highly sceptical.
5. The 200 patients who agreed to take part in the research trial, many of whom were highly sceptical.

Added together, these five different groups represent a total of a few thousand people. The similarity of comments made by the individuals in each of the groups further confirms the validity of the statements across all five categories.

For the benefit of patients, it is important to discover ways to maximize the potential of the placebo effect. Healers might well say that the placebo effect is the person's own self-healing ability in action. Yet the positive effects of healing on plants and animals demonstrate that a separate element is also at work, originating from an external source. Indeed, the researchers stated that the excellent results of our trial far exceed that which could be attributable to placebo alone.

Publication of the Research Paper

The quest to publish the research paper began towards the end of 2014. I had imagined that gaining publication would be reasonably straightforward; after all, the programme had been led by a university known for world-class research. Furthermore, its design and methodology had been given the seal of approval by a team of scientists appointed by the Lottery.

However, the editor of one prestigious, mainstream medical journal offered the following explanation for rejecting our paper:

> Your paper is not suitable for [our] readers [as they] do not subscribe to complementary medicine.

This reasoning seemed singularly unscientific. How can physicians make the decision whether or not to subscribe to a therapy if their journals will not publish research papers about them?

A repeated objection was that there was no placebo group to compare results with. Our research paper had detailed why it is not possible to provide a simulation for healing, but this was disregarded. It is worth noting that the same limitation applies to a number of medical interventions that have nevertheless been accepted in mainstream healthcare. Physiotherapy, for instance, cannot be faked.

It was decided that we would submit to a journal specializing in complementary medicine that offered open access. (The main medical journals only allow full access of the text to medical people and academics; ordinary members of the public usually only see the "abstract", a thumbnail sketch of the paper.) The full text would then be permanently available online for anyone to inspect.

The main, quantitative paper entitled "A pragmatic randomised controlled trial of healing therapy in a gastroenterology outpatient setting" was published in the *European Journal of Integrative Medicine*.[99]

The secondary, qualitative paper "Experiences of healing therapy in patients with irritable bowel syndrome and inflammatory bowel disease" was published in *BioMed Central Complementary Medicine and Therapies*.[100]

Within a few weeks of being available online, each paper was labelled on the respective journal's website as "Highly Accessed", confirming that they attracted a high level of interest.

Despite limitless online access, a research paper is still likely to attract fewer readers than a book. I therefore felt compelled to produce an easy-read version of the results, along with additional information that may inspire people to add healing to their healthcare provision.

Key Points

Quantitative Results

- The high level of recruitment achieved in a short period of time suggests that patients are keen to have healing, if offered within an NHS setting.
- The low level of drop-out suggests that patients enjoyed the sessions and felt that they benefited from them.
- No patient reported an adverse effect.
- Patients gained clinically significant improvements to their quality of life.
- Symptoms were alleviated.
- Five sessions incurred more benefit than fewer and those who had five sessions retained the benefits for longer.
- Some benefits continued to increase after their final healing session, and some benefits were maintained for at least 19 weeks.
- Some benefits had reduced by Week 24. This could be due to the well-known phenomenon that improvements eventually become the accepted norm. If so, all of the Week 24 figures reflect less than the actual degree of gains.
- The extent of improvement was deemed by our researchers to be greater than could be attributed to placebo.
- No individual or organization involved in this research stood to gain financially from its positive results, thereby adding further confidence to its findings.

Qualitative Results

- Participants described the experience of receiving healing as deeply relaxing and enjoyable.
- Many reported sensations while having healing that they had never experienced before when simply relaxing. Examples include warmth, energies, colours and upliftment.
- They felt an especially positive bond with the healer.
- They reported ongoing calmness and now being far less likely to worry.
- Many physical symptoms were alleviated.
- Sleep patterns had improved.

- A more positive frame of mind had emerged.
- Some reported using less medication.

Placebo Effect

- The placebo effect is a powerful ally for any practitioner, medical or otherwise.
- The hospital audit graphs reveal possible placebo improvements as a result of patients' consultations with Dr Singh. After a healing session, patients achieved further gains and to a substantial degree.
- If the placebo effect is deemed to be the sole cause of our research results, then healers must have learned how to harness its power.
- The mechanism that causes healing in animals, plants and cells in vitro (which cannot be placebo) must also benefit humans.

Conclusions

It would be logical to conduct trials that determine whether adding healing sessions to conventional care reduces NHS costs. It takes an inordinate length of time to secure funding, then conduct the trial and publish the research results. While waiting for such developments to occur, hospitals and doctors' surgeries could enlist healers (voluntary or paid) and conduct their own audits. They could then ascertain whether regular healing sessions help to reduce the number of appointments, medications and treatments required by their patients. A central register of such audits would facilitate sharing of the findings.

9

A Case Study

One of the people on the research trial, whose five sessions were all with me, kindly provided a written statement about his experience. After months of severe bowel problems, he was finally diagnosed with inflammatory bowel disease, specifically ulcerative colitis.

When a patient develops ulcerative colitis, the medical prognosis is that it will remain for life. In addition, the medicines available to alleviate the distressing and debilitating symptoms are not always effective.

Against this hopeless and depressing outlook, the account provided by this particular patient makes surprising reading. His professional career had been science-based, but he was open-minded when Dr Singh invited him to join the research programme. He was not one of the 22 people selected for interview.

> "Following bowel problems over the first six months of 2011, I underwent a colonoscopy at Good Hope Hospital and was diagnosed as having colitis. I was prescribed a specialist drug to help alleviate the symptoms and was then referred to Dr Singh's gastroenterology clinic at the hospital. The drug that I had been prescribed earlier made my symptoms worse, so it was changed to another. This second medication was no better than the first so it was changed again. The third medication was replaced with a fourth but still with no improvement. All of these drugs made my symptoms much worse and made me feel very ill. It became obvious that I was intolerant to all of the drugs that are normally used to help control colitis.
>
> "As the problems persisted I had consultations with Dr Singh's registrar, who explained to me that I may have to consider having my colon removed. During this distressing period I became depressed and irritable and my self-esteem was at an all-time low. Normality had gone out of my life. I did not go out very often and, when I did, I did not venture far from home because of my need to make regular visits to the bathroom. I was worried about having an 'accident' if I went out,

due to not getting to a toilet in time. I have never liked using public toilets and have always tried to avoid using them. This was a very difficult period for me and for my wife.

"During a further consultation with Dr Singh, who is someone I have great respect for, he suggested trying a different medication. He explained that it was not actually a drug, so I agreed to try it. He also asked me what I thought about alternative or complementary therapies. I told him that I was very open-minded about it as I had tried acupuncture on an old knee injury a few years before and this had been successful. He went on to explain about the research project being carried out with the University of Birmingham and Freshwinds and suggested that I might be a suitable patient to take part in the study.

"I started to take the new medication with no ill effects. My condition gradually started to improve and I was able to get out of the house more often. After 12 weeks, in April and May 2012, I received the course of five healing sessions with Sandy Edwards at Good Hope Hospital. I had no preconceived ideas or expectations of what might or might not happen. Throughout my working life I had dealt in facts. In my professional career, I had to make decisions based on factual evidence that was in my possession. Opinions and hearsay could not be considered.

"I like to research anything that I am involved in, whether it be hobbies, holidays or anything else. I like to make use of the information that is now so readily available through the internet. However, to allow me to be objective about the healing sessions, I felt that I should not research anything to do with healing or the research project. I wanted a clear, open mind with nothing to prompt me into thinking that changes, good or bad, were happening.

"At my first session with Sandy, she explained what she would do and made me feel at ease. I could hear everything that was going on around me, as you would expect from a busy hospital. However, following what Sandy was telling me, I became completely relaxed, and any noise or possible distraction drifted into the background.

"The first thing I noticed was that when Sandy touched my right shoulder I felt a very pleasant, warm feeling going right through my joint. [Unknown to Sandy] this joint had previously been injured, and it continued to be problematic and painful.

"As the session progressed, I had my eyes closed and started to see a purple flashing light which I can only describe as being like a beacon out at sea. This then gradually changed to a calming purple colour, just like purple silk. Throughout this time I was completely relaxed and pleasantly warm. It was like being in a calmer place. At the end of the session I felt completely different from when I had arrived. I was now warm and relaxed. A lot of my stress had gone.

"I continued with a further four sessions with Sandy and all were in a similar vein. I found them to be a pleasant experience, and my general demeanour and well-being improved enormously. I became less irritable and much calmer. My stress levels reduced considerably. I was beginning to cope with life better as my health improved. By this time I was going out more and able to cope better with the normalities of life. My wife told me that my whole demeanour had changed and that I was a lot easier to live with, a lot less grumpy. Certainly, we could go out socially more often.

"I had one major setback in July 2012 when we went away from home for the first time since being diagnosed with colitis [a year or so earlier]. We went to Southampton and stayed one night. I became very ill with sickness and diarrhoea, as bad as I have ever known. Later, at Dr Singh's clinic, it was thought that this was almost certainly food poisoning and not connected to colitis. However, this event made me lose all confidence in going away from home. Gradually, though, my confidence returned, and I have since had two small breaks away from home without problems.

"In October 2012 I underwent major surgery to have a replacement shoulder joint removed, and replaced with a 'reverse procedure'. This was a lengthy process that meant I took a lot of morphine and codeine to help with pain relief. Sleeping was quite difficult following the operation, but I found that, by using similar techniques to those during the healing sessions with Sandy, I was able to get myself into a calm and relaxed state, which helped me to sleep better.

"In conclusion, my life changed considerably in 2011 when I was diagnosed with colitis. I had only recently retired from work and I was suddenly restricted in what I was able to do and where I could go. I went through a dreadful period, which affected everything I did. My personality changed. I became very stressed and completely lacking in confidence.

"With the help and kindness of Dr Singh and Sandy Edwards I now have a great deal of normality back in my life. I am more confident, and my well-being has improved immensely. I am told that I am much easier to live with now, and I hope that I am able to continue like this into the future."

• • •

This man's testimony brings to life the practical meaning of some of the "statistically significant improvements" reported in the research paper. The figures suggest that a considerable proportion of the participants must have had similar experiences to these, which is heartening and uplifting. But, for this man, the story continued. When he returned for a subsequent appointment with Dr Singh, the following year, he welcomed the offer of a further healing session. He ultimately had a further five sessions with me during 2013, and I did not see him again until the following spring. He arrived full of smiles, and had this to say:

"After having had consultations with Dr Singh and healing sessions with Sandy Edwards, my health continued to steadily improve. My symptoms have now become minor in comparison to what I had been suffering before. For instance, simply leaving my house was difficult during the second part of 2010. But now my life has returned to a degree of normality.

"In July 2012 I had a setback when I became quite ill, but this was thought to be attributable to food poisoning. And in July 2013, I again had bowel problems that were quite bad. As I was about to go on holiday, my GP prescribed a course of steroid tablets, which helped to calm everything down and allowed me to travel. But other than these two episodes, my symptoms were generally improving.

"In September 2013 I was invited to take part in a routine bowel cancer screening programme for people my age. The results came back positive, meaning that something was wrong, including the possibility of cancer. I attended a consultation at University Hospital Coventry, where it was suggested that I consider having a colonoscopy to find out exactly what the problem was. I agreed that this would be the sensible course of action, but I was worried. Within a short period of time, the procedure was conducted, and I was verbally advised that there was no sign of ulcerative colitis in my bowel!

"I had been aware of continuous improvements to my symptoms, but to have this medical confirmation was totally unexpected and uplifting. I would have been ecstatic but for the possibility that cancer could not be ruled out until the polyps had been sent for examination. There were signs of diverticulosis, but this condition caused me hardly any problems in comparison to the dreadful time that I had gone through with ulcerative colitis.

"Some polyps were removed for further analysis, and it was a great relief to hear that these were free from cancer. The written report confirmed the verbal advice that I had been given: ulcerative colitis was not present in my bowel. This was, of course, very good news for me.

"I have continued to maintain stability with my bowels and colon, with only the occasional minor problem."

• • •

It was amazing to have medical confirmation that ulcerative colitis had completely disappeared. This is not possible to achieve by any medical intervention. By this time, the patient had received a total of ten healing sessions – five on the research trial and, six months later, an additional five at Dr Singh's clinic. But it is possible that the colitis disappeared before all ten sessions had been received.

Another unexpected benefit for this patient was regarding his replaced shoulder joint. A conventional shoulder replacement had proved unsuccessful, so he then had a "reverse" total shoulder replacement, in which the positions of the socket and metal ball are reversed. Despite this, the shoulder had remained very painful, with limited mobility and lack of power. Being right-handed, he found that his damaged right shoulder was making many normal activities very awkward, if not impossible. However, after the last healing session he was delighted to tell me that he had recently washed the car using his right hand for the first time. This was two years after the surgery.

In his younger days, this man had enjoyed playing contact sports. As a result, his ankles had suffered repeated injuries and were now usually painful. He told me that his ankles in particular always felt warm and comfortable during healing sessions, and that he could now walk more easily.

This man's life was being ruined by the debilitating and soul-destroying symptoms of ulcerative colitis. There is no hope of recovery from colitis, and he reacted badly to all the drugs offered. Then, after ten healing sessions, a thorough internal investigation showed no sign of ulcerative colitis. The last I heard, three years later, he continued to be entirely free of the disease.

As someone with a science-based career, he was mystified but enthralled by the sensations he experienced while receiving healing. He would usually have vivid images of his childhood and relive happy times with people who loved him.

In his statement he describes observing a purple light, pulsating like a beacon and dominating every session. Although I tell new patients that they might perceive colours, the only particular colour I mention is golden-white. I suggest they imagine themselves filled with this colour, simply to help them to relax; yet people often report afterwards that they actually saw purple. Purple has the shortest wavelength and the highest frequency of any colour that is visible to us. Hence, it is the last colour of the rainbow. Intriguingly, purple is the colour most associated with spiritual healing.

● ● ●

Despite the remarkable case study presented here, there is no guarantee that any number of healing sessions will eradicate colitis or any other condition. But there is nothing to lose by trying.

Cost/benefit issues are a primary factor for decision-making in the NHS. In today's money, the average medical expense of supporting each patient with ulcerative colitis has been estimated at £3,000 per year.[101] Add to this the potential cost of sick pay and benefit payments. Considering the overheads of maintaining just one individual throughout the remainder of their life, it must be worth considering options that have produced results like this.

Key Points

- Conventional treatments for this patient were ineffective.
- During a series of healing sessions, a complete and permanent recovery occurred despite the condition being considered incurable.
- A senior consultant physician witnessed the recovery.

10

What Next?

Ever-growing numbers of the British public were turning to complementary therapies, so the government conducted an in-depth investigation to assess whether this escalating situation should influence public
health policy. In 2000, the House of Lords conducted the inquiry, over-
seen by Lord Walton, a retired consultant neurologist who had once been
President of the British Medical Association.

During discussions, it transpired that various peers had experienced
complementary therapies and had benefited.

• • •

Lord Hodgson had been diagnosed with cancer, and underwent surgery
followed by six weeks of radiotherapy. Subsequent tests showed warning
signs of a recurrence, but no further treatments were possible, only
palliative care. Palliative care means medical care is limited to reducing
unpleasant symptoms. Like many others in this distressing and depressing
situation, he was prepared to cast around for unconventional options. He
was recommended to a particular reflexologist but was highly sceptical that
this could help. However, after a number of sessions he freely admitted
that it had been remarkably successful and that he felt better. He had to
pay for these treatments himself, and points out that taxpayers benefited
by his doing so, because the NHS was consequently saved the expense of
providing him with more pills and further appointments with the doctor.
Fellow patients also gained, because his appointments were now freed up
for them. By combining conventional treatments with a complementary
therapy he was able to resume a normal life. Lord Hodgson advocated that
the various disciplines should work in harmony with each other to relieve
the hard-pressed NHS, and to spread the burden of health provision that
is currently carried almost solely by orthodox physicians.

Lord Colwyn used kinesiology every day in his Harley Street dental
clinic as a diagnostic tool. He said that it worked brilliantly, but had no
idea why.[102]

• • •

As a young man, Lord Baldwin had damaged both knees in vigorous outdoor pursuits.[103] He was sent to specialists and then to two eminent physicians in Harley Street. The various treatments they administered proved fruitless.

Three years later, now hobbling around with knee bandages and a mindset of incurability, he was recommended to a spiritual healer in Cambridge. This healer spent half an hour waving his hands over the injured knees, all the while chatting about his job as a schoolteacher and his thoughts on politics. Lord Baldwin felt nothing, not even the sensation of heat or cold that he had been told to expect. He left in as much pain as when he arrived. But the next morning he was bewildered to find that the pain had vanished, and it was never to completely return.

Medical specialists had given him full care and attention over a period of three years, using the latest technology and knowledge. In contrast, the healer saw him in a back bedroom and spent 30 minutes on the job without concentrating on what he was doing.

Lord Baldwin makes the pertinent point that his recovery was unlikely to be due to the placebo effect because he fully expected results from the top professionals and had no faith at all in the healer.

• • •

Lord Rea, a retired GP, asserted that the common factor in many medical problems is stress, which can play a part in the origin or continuation of the physical condition.[104] Examples include migraine, asthma, irritable bowel syndrome, chronic joint pain, chronic back pain, chronic fatigue syndrome, eczema and allergies, HIV infection, multiple sclerosis, psoriasis, rheumatological conditions – all of which GPs find time-consuming and difficult to treat.

Many illnesses are a mystery to the scientific world. Research reveals that about two-thirds of all patients are suffering with long-term problems, and nobody knows why because no physical causes can be found by medical tests and investigations. For these people in particular, alternative ideas need to be explored.

• • •

The full Lords Report[105] was sent to the government, whose response was to agree that "there is scope for closer integration of CAM and conventional medicine in the interests of all relevant disciplines and, above all, in the interests of their patients. The Government recognises the need to develop the research capacity in this field."

Sufficient research was seen as a stumbling block, but it was revealed that only 8p was spent on CAM research for every £100 spent on researching orthodox methods.[106]

It was also suggested that conventional medical scientists and practitioners are inherently biased against CAM. Sir Iain Chalmers, of the Cochrane Collaboration, had this to say:

> *Many in the orthodox medical world remain either sceptical about the desirability of this trend [towards increasing use of CAM] or hostile to it. This scepticism seems to result partly from unwillingness within the orthodox mainstream to apply a single evidential standard when assessing the effects of healthcare.*

The latter sentence means that no matter how many individuals are seen to improve by using CAM therapies, the scientific community will not accept this as evidence. They will only accept placebo-controlled randomized control trials (RCTs). The limitations of RCTs were discussed earlier, and also why it is not possible to design a placebo for healing.

Before we began our RCT, Dr Singh warned me that even if the research trial were an outstanding success, the scientific community would merely add it to the body of evidence. It would not necessarily encourage the NHS to embrace or provide healing any more than it had done in the past. It was disappointing to think that the results of such a large and high-quality trial might not make the slightest impact on healthcare provision. If more evidence is needed, who is likely to pay for it? This one project cost £205,000 plus countless hours of goodwill. And who would go to the effort of applying for a grant to research healing when the odds of success in securing funding are so low?

This particular trial concentrated specifically on people with IBS and IBD, and the scientific community must surely now concede that healing has been found to be beneficial for these two conditions. However, they would not agree that healing could be considered helpful for any other disorder. According to the scientific world, healing trials would need to be conducted for every illness and ailment before it could be deemed beneficial for all of them. This would be impossible to achieve. Financially, it is out of the question, and who would undertake all those projects? It would be unrealistic to expect funding for even one additional trial of healing, let alone a myriad of them.

Of course, it is vital that pharmaceutical drugs be trialled for each separate illness they are designed to remedy before they can be prescribed. All drugs have side effects, and doctors and patients alike need to be confident that a new medication is likely to be efficacious and safe to take. For those taking multiple drugs for a variety of illnesses, the combination of chemical ingredients also needs to be considered.

But healing is different. Healing energy is not manufactured using specific ingredients for a particular purpose. It is simply a natural, wholesome energy that seems to find its own way to where it is needed most, no matter what the trouble is. Nor has any healing trial provided evidence of an adverse impact. The concerns that apply to the approval of pharmaceutical drugs are therefore not relevant to healing.

An abundance of examples has already been given to support the view that healing is efficacious for all kinds of conditions. The following series of evaluations, funded by the North Cumbria Health Authority, also bears this out.

An evaluation in 2004 involved 300 patients who, between them, had a wide range of ailments.[107] Each patient received four healing sessions within six weeks. The results showed that statistically and clinically significant improvements had been gained, both physically and psychologically. Gains included stress reduction, pain relief, increased ability to cope and increased general health. Results were $p < 0.0004$ for all symptoms, which means the odds against the changes being due to chance were four in 10,000 – very highly significant. The most substantial improvements were seen in those who had the worst symptoms to begin with.

Two further evaluations were funded jointly by the same health authority and Cumbria County Council. One involved 35 cancer patients,[108] while the other studied 147 people with mental health disorders.[109] As with the previous study, each patient received four healing sessions within six weeks and gained statistically significant results across a range of measures.

Added together, these three trials studied 482 patients, none of whom reported an adverse effect. As these three studies were preliminary evaluations, there was no control group. However, the positive outcomes illustrate the safety and effectiveness of healing. The results achieved were significant enough to convince the researchers that controlled trials should be conducted. However, I was unable to find evidence that subsequent trials had actually been instigated.

Additional studies have shown healing to help patients with mental health issues. A group of randomly assigned patients each received six weekly sessions. Significant improvements were gained regarding depression and stress, and benefits continued to be present one year later.[110]

Another trial involved 30 patients suffering from chronic pain, depression and sleep difficulties. They each received eight healing sessions, and gained significant improvements across all three aspects.[111]

A review in 2004[112] aimed to discover how effective healing was over a range of different conditions, including HIV, cancer and heart surgery. Over 30 trials were analyzed that met the researchers' standards. Although it was found that many of these studies were either poorly designed or poorly reported, they did indicate positive results. Outcomes such as reduced stress, anxiety and pain were commonly reported, as were physical improvements. Data showed that patients benefited emotionally, their relationships improved and they gained a greater sense of well-being. With no adverse side effects reported, the researchers concluded that healing is a safe and non-invasive therapy that should be researched further. They suggested that, if other research found similarly positive results, healing could be introduced alongside conventional healthcare so that lower medical costs could be achieved in respect of reduced drugs, shorter hospital stays and less clinic time.

Dr Michael Dixon has made healing available at his practice for decades. After regularly witnessing positive results, he conducted a study where 57 chronically ill patients each received ten weekly healing sessions.[113] The term "chronic" refers to any illness that has lasted for three months or more, but these patients had suffered for more than six months. They had failed to respond to any other approach, whether conventional or complementary. Two weeks after the healing sessions had been completed, 81 per cent of the treated group thought their symptoms had improved, and nearly half of these thought their improvements were substantial. Gains were still evident three months later.

In 2008, Dr Dixon and his partners created the Culm Valley Integrated Centre for Health, which is widely regarded as a prototype for general practice of the future and includes healing in its provision of care.

Dr Craig Brown conducted a similar study in his practice. 33 chronically ill patients received one 20-minute healing session every week for eight weeks. Using a comprehensive questionnaire, it was established that there were improvements in all measures of their quality of life, maintained for at least six months.[114]

All of the above evaluations, along with the many other trials referenced, serve to support the healing community's assertion that healing can help any condition. As mentioned before, if an inspection were carried out of the MYMOP data in our trial, it might reveal that a range of maladies had been alleviated during the course of our study, not just those associated with IBS and IBD.

Also, although our trial focused on IBS and IBD patients, the positive results are relevant to patients with other medical issues. Hippocrates (460–370 BC), the father of modern medicine, stated that "all disease begins in the gut". Although he was not entirely correct, modern studies suggest that this is true for many conditions. For instance, diet-induced inflammation can lead to type 2 diabetes, obesity, liver disease and many of the world's most serious diseases.[115] Due to the gut–brain axis, certain gut disorders are also linked to schizophrenia, autism, anxiety and depression.[116]

Regarding psychological problems, evidence has led researchers to conclude that most of the therapeutic change gained by counselling is due to the patient's own resources and their relationship with the practitioner. Their findings suggest that 15 per cent of any improvement is attributable to the placebo effect and another 15 per cent to the particular technique used. If only 15 per cent of the improvement is down to the technique, it makes sense to use the cheapest and quickest option that works.

Looking at the results of our research programme and the many other healing trials, plus my two hospital audits and hundreds of patients' comments, it is inevitable to conclude that healing helps the mind and the emotions. With sessions only taking 20 minutes, far more people can receive healing per hour than can be given counselling. This could speed up improvement time and reduce costs. In the event that there were patients who did not respond sufficiently to healing, they could then be referred to counselling.

Many of us know from our own personal experience that the mind and emotions play a part in the health of our physical body. In the Lords

Report, Professor Patrick Bateson (then Vice President of the Royal Society) states that psychological factors do affect physical health:

> When somebody suffers chronic stress, bereavement or loses a job ... they are much more prone to disease and more likely to get cancer, and it is now believed that this is because of suppression of the immune system, which is constantly cleaning up bacteria and viruses and also cleaning up cells that are cancerous.

• • •

Traditional science holds the materialist view that the mind is a product of the physical brain, despite masses of evidence that the mind affects the body. Scientific organizations that work to break through this limiting and erroneous barrier include The Galileo Commission, whose remit is:

> to find ways to expand science so that it can accommodate and explore important human experiences and questions that science, in its present form, is unable to integrate.

Following widespread consultation with 90 advisors representing 30 universities worldwide, they published the Galileo Commission Report entitled *Beyond a Materialist Worldview—Towards an Expanded Science*.[117]

The Research Council for Complementary Medicine exists to promote research that will widen the availability of, and access to, safe and effective complementary medicine for patients, to help prevent disease and improve patients' health and quality of life.[118]

The Institute of Noetic Sciences works to reveal the interconnected nature of reality through scientific exploration and personal discovery. Their scientists apply the rigours of their respective disciplines to explore common but extraordinary phenomena that are not yet understood, which naturally incorporates spirituality and healing.[119]

• • •

Returning to the Cumbrian studies involving people with mental health issues, the results of our trial confirmed their findings in that healing brought patients upliftment in the longer term. The general trend was that our patients worried less or felt emotionally better for months after their final healing session, and to a substantial degree. People tend to believe that their general level of happiness is set in stone because that is how they have always been. A number of people have labelled themselves as "a born worrier" and say they could never change. But research shows that this notion is a fallacy.

Measuring brain activity on an fMRI scanner reveals that when people are in a positive mood, the left prefrontal cortex lights up more than the right. Each time this activity occurs, physical changes take place in the brain that reset the person's general emotional state to a more uplifted level.[120]

For many years, I have encouraged people to imagine that positive thoughts and feelings strengthen the part of the brain that delivers happiness – the stronger that part is, the more capacity it has. It made sense to me that the brain would be like the physical body. Exercise a particular part regularly and it can do more for you. Who has not heard of the adage "use it or lose it"? It was wonderful to find that an element of this idea has been scientifically proven. These physical changes that occur in the brain could be the reason why the results of our trial revealed that benefits were sustained for months after the final healing session. Our study was limited to six months, but these improvements could be permanent for all we know.

As healers, we see evidence of this time and again because patients who have regular sessions usually become progressively more buoyant. Moreover, it would appear that a sufficiently intense burst of positive emotion must be able to make an immediate and permanent change, as demonstrated by the youngster featured in The Grand Round section. I have also maintained that the more contented and happy we are, the more physically healthy our body will be. It transpires that scientific evidence exists to support this hypothesis, too.

In 2011, Ed Diener of the University of Illinois led a review of more than 160 studies of human and animal subjects and found compelling evidence that happy people and contented animals tend to be healthier and live longer.[121] There were a few exceptions, but the overwhelming majority of the studies found that anxiety, depression, a lack of enjoyment of daily activities and pessimism were associated with higher rates of disease and a shorter lifespan. One of the studies followed nearly 5,000 university students for more than 40 years and found that those who were most pessimistic as students tended to die younger than their peers.

Animal studies, too, reveal a strong link between stress and poor health. Stressed animals, such as those living in crowded conditions, are more susceptible to heart disease, have weaker immune systems and tend to die younger. Laboratory experiments on humans have found that positive moods reduce the level of hormones related to stress, strengthen the immune system and speed the body's recovery after exertion. Other studies showed that hostilities between couples are linked to slow recovery from wounds and a weaker immune system.

Diener was surprised that the data across such a range of studies were so consistent. He reached the conclusion that government health recommendations – which currently focus on obesity, diet, smoking and exercise – should also include happiness.

Our study, along with many others referenced in this book, shows that healing sessions engender a more uplifted mood. People can test whether this is true, and whether it does lead to improved health, by utilizing MYMOP questionnaires. Measuring changes each week, over a course of regular healing sessions, will answer the question. Naturally, if benefits were noted and were continuing, there would be no reason to stop the experiment.

Plotting progress on paper is highly valuable because people soon forget how acutely they previously suffered from a particular ailment and in how many ways it had affected their lives.

A completed set of forms would provide persuasive evidence to convey to a physician the ways in which healing had been beneficial. People normally only go to see their doctor when they are unwell. Hardly anyone makes an appointment to report that they have recovered. If it were difficult to speak to the doctor or consultant personally, a copy of the completed forms could be delivered to the doctor's office or hospital along with a covering letter.

As mentioned earlier, scientists would contend that the positive results of our healing trial are only relevant to people with IBS or IBD. However, there were some individuals within the trial who said that their symptoms did not improve yet the quality of their life was enhanced. After having healing sessions, they could cope with their illness better and had a more positive frame of mind. This uplift continued until at least Week 24. If an enhanced quality of life can be gained regardless of symptoms, then it follows that healing must be valuable for patients with any other condition.

People come along to our healing centre with all kinds of problems, and their feedback is in line with everything in this book. Those afflicted with disease, illness, skin conditions, insomnia and physical injuries have been helped. So, too, have people suffering from pain, fear, anxiety, bereavement, depression, stress, loneliness, anger and resentment. Some have been astonished at the change in themselves. Multitudes of healers across the country and around the world repeatedly receive similar feedback from their own patients.

Another effect of healing that people rarely notice, unless specifically asked, is that their eyesight has improved. This corresponds with the findings of Dr William H. Bates (1860–1931), who asserted that relaxation is the key to better vision. Through his work as a well-respected eye surgeon and a tutor of ophthalmology at the New York Medical School, he came to question the prevailing theories and practices. It was accepted then – as it mostly is now – that prescription glasses were the only answer to long- or short-sightedness. Bates gave up his lucrative practice to conduct research at Columbia University and many of his papers were published by the *New York Medical Journal*. His findings indicated that eyesight varies tremendously according to someone's emotional state. This was consistent with previous trials showing that people tend to become short-sighted when they feel apprehensive. Bates himself was long sighted but, by developing ways to avoid straining his eyes when reading, he regained normal vision.

Nowadays, the Bates Method is often associated with doing eye exercises but, in reality, he recommended using relaxed natural vision habits all day long. He made it a life's work to bring this message to the masses, and his teachings are available to download free of charge from the internet.[122]

The most remarkable experience I have witnessed regarding vision improvement was with a woman who was virtually blind without her glasses. She took them off to have a healing session and relaxed for the next 20 minutes. When she opened her eyes afterwards, she looked around the room, blinking with astonishment. Not only could she see everything clearly, but the colours were very much brighter. Having worn glasses since childhood, she could not contemplate being without them, not even for a short while to see how long this improvement might last. She slipped them back on and had to wait for a few minutes while her eyes adjusted to the strength of the spectacles.

Although I do not need glasses, I had a similar experience myself. While coming out of a deep meditation, I opened my eyes prematurely and discovered that I could read the text of an open book about 20 metres away. As I returned to normal consciousness, the far-away text became increasingly blurred, as did the book, until my usual standard of vision returned.

These two cases identify that we each, temporarily, had the ability to see far better than we normally do. Both of us must therefore have the necessary anatomical equipment to do so. Something must be negatively affecting how those physical parts work when we are going about our normal day. Stress seems the likely culprit since it causes tension in the body's muscles, which probably includes the eye muscles. If so, either the relaxation techniques taught by Bates, or the stress relief brought about by healing, could be expected to have a positive effect on eyesight. People can test this hypothesis for themselves by using either of these two methods and plotting weekly progress by using an eyesight test chart.

As regards any side effects of healing, nothing detrimental was reported by any of the people in my two hospital audits or the research trial. Allowing for the few individuals in my audits whom I may have seen more than once, this makes a total of around 450 hospital patients who were not harmed in any way. We could add to this figure the hundreds of other hospital patients who received healing at Dr Singh's clinic, the medical professionals at the Nursing in Practice exhibitions and the people who have flowed through our voluntary healing centre.

In cases where conventional healthcare is unable to help patients, it has to be more cost-effective for the NHS to provide complementary therapies that have been shown to be beneficial.[123] Additional treatment strategies that are effective would be highly desirable for these patients. Researchers on a different trial made the following statement:

> Conventional drugs are aimed at suppressing symptoms, but we are now much more aware that symptom management is not limited only to the prescription of drugs.[124]

Our own researchers made the following recommendation in our paper:

> Further cost-effectiveness evaluation is required before determining the role healing therapy may play in resource-restricted health

services, but patients with IBS and IBD seen in secondary care, who remain symptomatic despite best medical care, should be considered for healing therapy ...

• • •

The results of our trial will be especially welcomed by healers and healing organizations whose valuable work might now hope to receive greater acceptance by the medical world. Doctors are busy, time is short and resources are stretched, so it would seem ideal to have mainstream healthcare supported by healing and by other complementary therapies that have been similarly trialled and proven to be safe and effective.

The introduction of complementary therapies to standard healthcare provision would be a popular move, welcomed by many patients. As mentioned before, three quarters of the people asked were in favour of complementary therapies being made widely available on the NHS.[125] In 2004, it was found that around 10 per cent of the UK adult population had accessed a complementary therapy during the previous year[126] and, in the main, they did so to supplement their conventional care.[127] This illustrates the fact that a great number of people are keen to find effective complementary remedies to assist their recovery and help them resume a normal life.

The term "healing therapy" can include any one of an array of healing methods and practices, with training standards ranging from scant to professional. This is why the research paper and my book have underlined the importance of using properly trained healers who belong to a reputable organization.

Also, when practitioners belong to a reputable association, they are bound by a professional code of conduct, which protects the public in two ways. First, individuals with unwholesome intentions are more likely to be deterred from joining an organization with proper standards in place. Second, any unprofessional behaviour can be reported to the organization so that an investigation can be instigated, and disciplinary procedures applied. The following example illustrates the point.

Angie Buxton-King describes in her book *The NHS Healer* a desolate time in her life when she sought healing. Her young son had died of cancer. After several uplifting and beneficial sessions with a private healer, he advised her that the only way to resolve her remaining problems was to have sex with him. Outraged that someone in a position of trust could attempt to groom and violate a vulnerable person, she sought to report him. But he did not belong to any organization, and she was therefore powerless to stop him practising. It is important to check that a healer belongs to a reputable association, and any respectable practitioner will gladly provide evidence of their membership.

Besides a strict code of conduct, the Healing Trust employs additional methods to ensure that applicants are genuine and upstanding. Personal references, tutors and mentors all play a part. At the same time, though, every effort is made to welcome sincere applicants and to support their development.

Although the research trial only included healers taught by the Healing Trust, similar results are achieved by equally well-trained healers from other organizations. Voluntary healing groups and private healers can be found via the organizations listed on page 228. The level of fee charged has no correlation to their ability as a healer. Many excellent healers are volunteers and, for various reasons, it suits some of them to work outside of their own home and as part of a voluntary group.

The prospect of going to a healing centre for the first time may feel unsettling, but healers are invariably warm and welcoming. One of the many benefits of going to a centre is that patients can try different healers to see if the experience varies. In the unlikely event that a patient feels uneasy with a particular healer, they can simply ask to see someone else. Also, if a patient's preferred healer is absent there will probably be another available, so sessions need not be missed. When away from home, whether holidaying or working, it may be possible to find a healing centre nearby. And, financially, voluntary healing centres are very accessible as they usually suggest a minimum donation of a nominal amount, or nothing at all for those who cannot afford to contribute.

Sessions with a private healer might cost more but they are ideal for patients who do not want others to know that they are having healing. They are assured of having the same healer every time, and they may feel that they can relax better in a private treatment room.

Another avenue through which regular healing can be made available is at support groups, like the MND and breast cancer meetings mentioned earlier. One has to stand back and admire the indomitable spirit of the people who organize these groups and the people who attend them. Strange as it may seem, humour manages to survive, even within groups that support the most distressing and life-limiting diseases. One example is that of a bowel cancer group that has named itself The Semi-Colons! The various self-help groups that our healers have attended have been fun as well as rewarding, and I would encourage anyone to take advantage of this form of support. On the financial side, when volunteers attend such groups, attendees receive healing free of charge, and their organization usually makes a donation to the healing group.

People sometimes need a course of regular sessions before they can detect a change and, even then, some are oblivious to their own improvements and it is only when their family and friends pass comment that they realize they have benefited. When I first had healing, long before I trained, it was only after six weekly sessions that I realized the profound difference that healing had made to me. I was sleeping better, laughing more and responding to situations in a much more positive way.

The physical problem for which I had sought healing – psoriasis – did improve, but not by much. The most incredible revelation was that a lifetime fear had dissolved. I had always been afraid of being alone in a house at night. Strangely, I was fine outdoors in the dark at any time, but not inside a house. I have no idea why. Logic told me that thousands of nights of my life had passed without incident, so why should this particular night be any different? But emotions are far more powerful than reason and, regardless of the sense of it, I hardly slept whenever my husband went away on occasional business trips. After a handful of healing sessions, I noticed the amazing difference within myself and began to revel in having the place to myself on those occasions. I did not wish my husband to be away but, when he had to be, it felt liberating to be able to do what I liked, when I liked. Of course, I still had the children to care for and a business to run, but this new sense of freedom and confidence was exhilarating. My husband continued to go away on business, but my response to his short absences was now entirely positive. Nothing had changed in my life, only my reaction to it.

This deeply held fear had been dissolved without my needing to realize it was there. I did not need to remember that it existed. Nor did I need to unearth what had caused it in the first place. These observations contribute towards why I think it is unnecessary for a healer to quiz patients about what is troubling them. My own personal experience illustrates how hidden, underlying fears can melt away to make room for a more confident and buoyant mindset.

Likewise, the patients involved in the research programme may have found that issues unrelated to IBS or IBD had been resolved. Perhaps health questionnaires should include a section that identifies and measures fears

Whether people choose to have healing sessions or not, there is plenty that they can do for themselves. Quick and simple techniques have helped people to alleviate pain, gain peace of mind and improve their health. Some of the patients referred to earlier have been amazed at what they could do for themselves. The following account relates an experience of my own.

Out of the blue, I began having spasmodic stabbing pains in the abdomen that were so severe that they made me cry out each time they struck. There was no telling when an episode might start or subside but they were most often during the night. No amount of painkillers made a difference, and two courses of antibiotics were ineffective. Preliminary investigations revealed nothing, and the next step was to have a scan. If someone else had been in this predicament, I would have offered healing at the outset. For myself, the thought did not cross my mind. Not until I was doubled up one night, in the thick of yet another bout, did it occur to me. When I focused on healing the very core of the pain, it melted away within two seconds – literally – and never returned. Despite having seen this happen for many patients, I was incredulous when it worked for me. Now I could identify with the bewilderment and sense of disbelief that so many of my patients had expressed. Thank goodness I had discovered healer training years ago. For those who are interested, the quick technique I used is outlined on page 226.

As my own example demonstrates, I readily reach for the medicine cabinet at the first sign of pain or discomfort. Like many others, I may try natural remedies first, but if that does not work quickly enough, my next stop is the chemist or the doctor's office. I have no intention of suffering if there is a pill or procedure that will bring swift relief and allow me to go about my normal day. We are extremely fortunate in the UK to have access to dedicated medical professionals free of charge and a plethora of pharmaceutical drugs at minimal cost. But, as our trial and many others confirm, this indispensable medical care can be further enhanced by the provision of healing, especially in situations where conventional treatment is ineffective or causes side effects. The next question is whether members of the public are likely to seek healing independently.

Since the completion of our trial, Dr Singh has seen a number of the participants at their follow-up appointments. They have told him how much they enjoyed the sessions and that they had benefited from the experience, but they would not consider having healing outside of the NHS. It gave them confidence to know that the particular healer had been approved by the hospital and that the therapy had been recommended by the consultant. They felt protected by being treated in a medical setting. Clearly, many more people would be likely to take advantage of healing if it were made available in doctors' surgeries and hospitals.

It would also be more readily taken up if it were free, of course. Citizens of the UK are accustomed to receiving healthcare without being charged and there may be a psychological barrier against having to pay. Some people might baulk at the idea of even a nominal fee to receive healing at a hospital. Others simply could not afford the additional outlay.

To be made available on the National Health Service (NHS), each medicine and treatment has to be approved by the National Institute for Health and Care Excellence (NICE). NICE looks to see how well a medicine or treatment works in relation to how much it costs, to ensure the NHS gets value for money. The NHS is legally obliged to fund any treatments recommended by NICE. The Medicines Act 1968 provides that a new medicine can receive a marketing authorization from NICE if it is marginally more effective than a placebo.[128] It does not have to be more effective than existing and well-established medicines.

The British Medical Association defines complementary therapies as "those that can work alongside conventional medicine", which implies tacit approval of spiritual healing. Our trial demonstrates how easy it is to provide spiritual healing in a medical environment, and the benefit to patients above and beyond best medical care.

On the face of it, then, it should be a straightforward matter for healing to be made available on the NHS, and for a range of medical conditions.

Until that day comes, what can each of us do to encourage doctors and hospitals to make healing available?

The first thing is to make the results of our research trial known to people in key positions, both nationally and locally. This includes doctors and consultants, hospitals, primary care trusts, NHS chiefs, healthcare administrators, government officials, MPs and local councillors. If people in influential positions learn how patients have been helped by healing, they may take steps to make it available at NHS sites. Some surgeries might take the pragmatic view – as Cleveland Clinic did (page 24) – that it is worth implementing a cost-efficient therapy that has been shown to be safe and effective.

Second, people who have benefited from healing need to tell their doctor or specialist about their experience. A completed set of weekly questionnaires would give impressive evidence that may encourage a doctor to be more open-minded towards healing. As a result, a doctor's office or a hospital might consider trialling a healer, either paid or unpaid. There is no reason why a voluntary healing group should not be based at an NHS venue if space is available.

Third, and vitally important, is to broadcast to the public the fact that healing exists. The news of our research trial would be very useful but, mentioned before, not many people read research papers so I felt driven to write a book about it. Initially, I could only self-publish because I could not divulge the research results to a publisher prior to the research papers appearing in medical journals. As soon as they did, I made my book available on Amazon, set up a Facebook page, launched my website, and sent out a raft of emails.

My efforts to gain media coverage for the research results bore some fruit.

BBC News *Midlands Today* – which has a primetime slot – returned to the hospital and filmed Dr Singh, a patient and me. Sadly, their TV programme did not convey how outstanding the results are, but the film crew must have been impressed because they asked for a fistful of healing leaflets to distribute back at the studios. The BBC website also carries the story.[129]

Film-maker Dena Barnett brought a film crew from London to interview Dr Singh, a patient and me at the hospital. It was the final shoot for her documentary *Spiritual Healing: A New Frontier*.[130]

A German film-maker interviewed me for his feature film *Self Healed*,[131] initially released in German with plans for many languages. It features the well-known scientist and author Rupert Sheldrake, along with an impressive line-up of 19 other scientists, medical doctors and healers.

• • •

It was an unexpected delight to receive an invitation to present the research results at the Houses of Parliament in London. The meeting was arranged by the All-Party Parliamentary Group for Integrated Healthcare, and I was their only speaker. Around 60 people battled atrocious weather that evening to listen to my talk, and according to a member of the Group, the audience was "fired up" by it. It would be a tremendous breakthrough if this helped gain UK government attention and contributed to bringing healing into the NHS.

Also encouraging was a very positive review of my book by the Royal College of Nursing in their magazine, which reaches 96,000 nurses.

Substantial and highly supportive reviews and articles have also appeared in international online publications including the Scientific & Medical Network's journal *The Paradigm Explorer* as well as *Complementary Medicine Research*, *Positive Health Online* and *Kindred Spirit*.

Nexus, an Australian magazine with a worldwide following, printed a two-page article, with a highlight on the front cover.

The famous and fascinating Watkins bookstore in London allowed me to give a talk there, and also printed a two-page article in their prestigious magazine.

The Society for Psychical Research reviewed my book for their members and also invited me to give a further talk in London.

Lynne McTaggart's online magazine *What Doctors Don't Tell You* printed an article and interviewed me online. They offered me a stand at their inaugural Get Well Show at Olympia, London, where I also gave a presentation of the research results. The three-day show was vibrantly successful, and is expected to be an annual event in London and Los Angeles.

German publishers Kopp Verlag heard of my book and offered me a publishing deal for the German-language edition. I was thrilled to accept, and – incredibly – they sold nearly 1,800 hardback copies in the first nine weeks. It was news of their success that led to the exciting worldwide (except German) deal that I now have. Intriguingly, this publishing offer arrived halfway through Healing Awareness Week, on the day of a full Super Moon that was travelling through my birth sign!

Personal accounts convey the real difference that healing can make to an individual's life. It takes courage to offer one's own story to the media, but such articles are engaging, they instil hope, and they inspire others to take that first step. If different people's stories were regularly aired on television and radio programmes, and published in newspapers and magazines, it would help raise awareness and create interest. Healing could be mentioned within the dialogue of films, woven into the storyline of TV dramas, incorporated within the lyrics of songs, and could be a topic included in chat shows and interviews.

Take, for instance, the television show in which Piers Morgan interviewed Michael Flatley of Riverdance fame. Morgan asked about a period of time when Flatley was ill for three years with a mystery virus. Dozens of top specialists were unable to discover what was causing the problem. Flatley became so badly affected that he was unable to leave the house for nearly a year. Sometimes, he could not coordinate himself enough to answer a simple question, no matter how hard he tried. Eventually, a member of his staff suggested that he see a particular healer in Ireland, and he agreed without hesitation. After the first session he went for a mile-long walk. After ten sessions he was dancing again.[132]

World champion snooker player Peter Ebdon was interviewed on BBC radio when he retired prematurely from the sport. After 29 years of wear and tear, he had developed physical problems in his back, neck and shoulder, causing excruciating pain. Painkillers made no difference, and the only other medical offering was an operation that carried with it the risk of paralysis. However, he discovered that spiritual healing and acupuncture reduced the pain considerably. He was so impressed by the range of improvements that he trained to be a professional healer with the College of Healing.[133]

If stories like these were to be discussed more frequently within the public domain, healing would gain greater acceptance.

To help bring more case studies into the public arena, my website can be used as a hub. Members of the public are invited to send me their stories, and journalists are encouraged to register their interest. I can then attempt to put appropriate parties in touch with each other. For those wishing to remain anonymous, their accounts can be included in my next book. To facilitate making these books accessible to more people, readers can ask their local lending library to stock a copy.

Also, thanks to the miracle of today's technology, any one of us can spend just a few minutes tapping on a computer to circulate healing stories to friends and other contacts all around the world.

Some people are afraid to tell their own friends about their healing experience, never mind taking it into the public domain. Fear of ridicule and criticism causes them to keep any unusual knowledge to themselves. But with thousands of healers in the UK, there must be a myriad of uplifting and inspiring stories being kept secret. If everyone felt free to talk openly about their experiences, it would soon become clear just how prevalent healing really is. Here are a few recent examples.

I gave two healing sessions to a woman with a heart problem, and we plan more when time allows. Perhaps her insightful and eloquent description will encourage others to consider having healing:

"For me, the most beautiful part about receiving healing is that there is no requirement for a case history; that painful unloading of one's baggage onto a desk in the clear light of day, which gets more boring every time I have to do it. Both healer and recipient come together in an attitude of openness, and an acceptance that whatever needs attending to will be attended to, without any copious note-taking. As someone who has unwillingly spent a lot of time in such an environment, I can say it's incredibly liberating to be taken at face value rather than as a collection of medical measurements and notes.

"You can imagine, then, it was a relief to be told that my job was just to relax in a nice comfy chair. I had arrived at my appointment like a coiled spring – fresh from a stressful day! and with my heart thumping fit to explode out of my chest. All other non-medical attempts to correct my irregular and very fast heartbeat had failed and this was literally my last port of call before going down the drug route. There was a lot at stake.

"After a short chat about how we'd proceed, Sandy stood a little way behind me and with carefully chosen words – very different from the 'relax your fingers, relax your hands,' approach – started talking me down from my pinnacle of stress. After filling my head with beautiful images of lightness and well-being, she stepped towards me, bringing her hands around each side of my head. Then with a snap of her fingers she abruptly moved back again, and said that I needed to give permission for the healing to take place – permission to allow myself to receive it – which was interesting. I wondered what I would need to let go of in order to do so.

"Sandy stepped back in again and with my eyes closed I became

aware of a deep and gentle heat within my body as she recommenced the healing. It was like standing under a heat lamp, but so much more powerful – the warmth worked its way down into the deepest levels of my stress, unknotting muscles and fibros as it did so, especially in my stomach. I discovered there were tensions that didn't want to release and as the warmth worked its magic I fought the urge to resist. As I did so, great tides of emotion rose up and threatened to swamp me, as they so often do when I try to relax. It's a family joke that I can cry at anything, but to be honest, it's really exhausting and I wish I didn't. My habit has always been to tighten my throat and choke the tears back, but Sandy had earlier suggested that I allow the feelings to silently arise and breathe them out through a gently open mouth. I managed to do this, but with tears streaming down my face. It was so good to just let go. The problem with an irregular heartbeat is that the very fact it is irregular causes a certain level of tension, which leads to more stress, so I was getting into a vicious circle that even my regular periods of meditation couldn't untangle. As the intensity of the heat gradually lessened, Sandy finished the healing and by the time she moved away I was more relaxed than I'd been for a very long time. It took several moments to come back to my body and the room, and when I finally – and somewhat grudgingly! – opened my eyes it felt as though the coat hanger had been taken away from my shoulders and I was facing the world from a new perspective.

"The sense of deep peace and relaxation lasted for several days – during which time I sent Sandy a message saying that I was sleeping well and that I was feeling more human than I had done for ages. My heartbeat was still irregular, but I at least managed to have a couple of walks, which is something else I hadn't been able to do for a while. From the medical viewpoint the problem hasn't been resolved yet, I am beginning to feel that at another level some much deeper healing is being facilitated, and the strands are slowly becoming untangled."

• • •

It was interesting to read that I snapped my fingers. In reality, she had heard the strange clicks in my fingertips, described earlier, that convey to me that I should continue healing there.

A friend we see each year on holiday told me that his palms had become so painful that his consultant had proposed surgery on both hands. He was shown the scans, which revealed the physical damage inside that was causing the pain. Being cautious, he agreed to only his right hand being treated – and lucky he did because afterwards it was worse than before. I offered healing sessions but he rolled his eyes in dismissal and shook his head. His wife nudged him to agree but he resisted. When I demanded – with a twinkle – to know what he was afraid of, he threw up his hands and capitulated.

He thoroughly enjoyed receiving healing and, after the first session, had to admit that the pain had reduced. After the second session, a week later, he announced that he had no further need for healing because he could manage with the low-level discomfort that remained. I pressed him to continue having sessions until the pain had completely gone. After just one more session, the pain disappeared completely and both hands have remained so ever since. He related his experience to many of his friends, one of whom had difficulty walking due to a heart condition. After a few sessions, he outpaced his wife!

Another had been poisoned by chemicals 20 years earlier and, since then, he had suffered terrible pains and cramps many times a day in random parts of his body. During the first session, he was astonished to feel energies coursing through his body. Each week he noticed improvements, and after a few sessions he was delighted to report having had only one short bout of pain in ten days. We shall resume sessions when we holiday there again next year.

A lady with intense pain and mobility issues experienced healing for the first time. She reported major improvements in hip pain and wrote:

> The combination of the heat from [Sandy's] hands and her calming voice, for someone as highly stressed as me, created a very serene experience that left me feeling rejuvenated for days. Anybody who has not had healing before should keep an open mind and try it.

• • •

I asked Balens Insurance, market leaders in the field of insuring complementary therapists, how many healers there might currently be in the UK. They confirmed that they have 80,000 therapist clients but were unable to say how many of these were healers. However, they had an interesting story about how they came to specialize in complementary-therapy insurance.

Balens was originally a general commercial brokerage but three generations on, David Balen became involved in the family business. As a young man, he had backpacked around India and contracted hepatitis A. He became gravely ill and, during the process of recovery, he learned of complementary therapies from fellow travellers. He benefited from this knowledge, and the experience broadened his view of health.

A few years later, he had a serious accident. His injuries were incorrectly treated by the NHS, resulting in long-term complications that caused him trauma and pain for many years. He turned again to natural therapies, which he believes sustained him throughout the ordeal and led to his recovery.

In 1990, colleagues in the therapy world asked David to help with developing professional insurance cover for therapists. Balens was the first company to offer this standard of cover, and they clearly paved the way for others in the industry to follow. Their figure of 80,000, together with a survey suggesting that 40 per cent of all CAM practitioners are healers,[134] points to around 32,000 healers on Balens' books, plus all those who are covered by other insurers.

This must mean that a tremendous number of people have received healing. If everyone talked openly about their experience, a growing number of others would surely be more likely to seek healing. Of the many people who benefit from healing, some subsequently feel inspired to help others in the same way. And if more people received healing, we would eventually have more healers. This can only be a good thing – so long as they are properly trained.

People are often sceptical that they could become a healer, but I believe that anyone can if they are determined. Various signs can indicate a natural ability, such as tingling in the hands when the person thinks about healing. Some people have an obvious natural ability but cannot accept that it is real. Someone once told me about various occasions when she had placed her hands on ailing friends who then improved instantly. Despite the repeated evidence, it was too unbelievable for her, and she continues to doubt her ability. Mixing with other healers would help her gain confidence and to acknowledge her gift. Proper training would ensure that she was not depleting herself when giving healing, and would also maximize the beneficial effects.

For those wishing to train, calling in at a voluntary healing centre is a good first step. Visitors can have a relaxed chat with the healers, view a session in progress and experience a healing session themselves.

Some people only ever intend to give healing quietly to family and friends, in which case the initial training courses give sufficient knowledge. However, almost all students find training to be so enriching that they are eager to enrol for the next level. Good quality training offers a firm foundation for dealing with one's own life challenges as well as for supporting loved ones through theirs. Life events will still occur, but our response to them is liable to be more constructive.

As additional people train to become healers and healing becomes more prevalent, the effects can only be increasingly better for the health and well-being of society as a whole.

Most people are keen to have a long, happy and healthy life. Scores of studies carried out since the 1980s suggest that people who follow some sort of spiritual path fare better than those who do not. Dr H. Koenig of Duke University aggregated 3,300 of these papers and the findings indicated a clear set of benefits. These covered physical and mental health, general well-being and the wider community.[135] These people seem to recover from major surgical procedures better and they have a lower incidence of nearly all the major diseases, including heart disease and cancer. According to some surveys, they live longer by seven to 13 years.[136] With traditional church attendance in steep decline, regular healing sessions could provide the spiritual element that is missing from so many people's lives.

Very often, people seek healing as a last resort when there seems to be no other option. They have either suffered for a long time or they have had a bolt out of the blue – for example a heart attack – that has shaken them to their roots. We often do not realize how much our thoughts and actions affect our bodies until something suddenly goes wrong with our health and we have to re-evaluate our lifestyle and priorities. But there is no need to wait until something drastic develops. It is far better to recognize a small health issue as being a nudge to find healing. We shall have this same body until we die, so it is in our own interest to make it last and wear well. And since it is our closest friend and lifetime companion, it makes sense to treat it as a precious gift and have a great relationship with it.

Healing has been shown to generate health, happiness and hope, with no adverse side effects. The next logical step is to take a slice of this action for ourselves. Now is the best time to make that happen. Delay simply puts off the moment when improvements can begin. The more we benefit physically and emotionally, the better it is for ourselves, for our loved ones and for everyone with whom we come into contact. No matter how well and happy we think we are, nobody is physically perfect and totally stress-free.

If the answer to any of the following questions is "no", healing sessions can improve your life.

1. Is your body in good shape and in perfect health?
2. Do you feel fulfilled and happy with life?
3. Do you have good relationships with everyone you know?
4. Do you feel guilty about anything?
5. Do you sleep well?
6. Do you approve of yourself?

If the answer to any of the following questions is "yes", healing can help you.

1. Do you have any fears or phobias?
2. Are you allergic to anything?
3. Do you take medication for anything?
4. Do you have any addictions?
5. Do you get stressed?
6. Do you get irritated or annoyed?
7. Are you harbouring a grudge against anyone?
8. Do you worry?

Honest answers to the above reveal that we all have something worthwhile to gain from healing. Healing sessions must be the easiest and most pleasant way to achieve improvements in all of these areas and more. If you still cannot believe that healing can help, be scientific and try it for yourself. Using your choice of questionnaires and following the simple guidance provided, you can plot your own progress over a series of six weekly sessions. If you notice any benefit from these six treatments, it makes sense to carry on.

Fear, anxiety, worry, depression, stress and anger are just a few examples of the inward-looking emotions that weigh us down and hold us back. Left unchecked, they cause us physical harm, according to scientific evidence. The sooner we upcycle the energy of destructive thoughts and emotions, the more we can enjoy the remainder of our lives. Everyone around us benefits, especially our children and our grand-children. People repeatedly experience healing as a relaxing method of transforming physical pain and unhelpful emotions into calmness, vitality and improved health. You could be one of them.

But what if you cannot find a local healer? Then self-healing is the answer, and we shall be taking a look at this in the next chapter.

Key Points

Benefit of Healing Sessions

- Clinical trials have shown healing to be beneficial for a wide range of conditions – physical, mental and emotional.
- After receiving healing many patients have reported improvements including pain relief, reduced symptoms, increased mobility, reduced addictions, reduced stress, reduced fears and phobias, reduced anxiety and worry, increased confidence and motivation, improved sleep and improved relationships.
- Since gut disorders are the root cause of other physical and psychological problems, the results of our trial have been found to be relevant to a host of other patients.
- Healing sessions engender an uplifted state of mind, which is synonymous with happiness. The sensation of happiness causes physical changes in the brain that can be permanent. Happy people have been found to be healthier and live longer.
- People with a spiritual element in their lives have been found to be healthier and live longer. Healing sessions provide a spiritual element.

Healing Within Medical Establishments

- Healing sessions are as effective as some medical treatments but at a fraction of their cost.
- Healing sessions can be beneficial for conditions where medical treatments are ineffective.
- Healing is likely to cost the least of any complementary therapies,

because no equipment or supplies are needed and it takes the shortest time to conduct a session.

- Healing is the most universally usable therapy to adopt, as it does not involve physical touch or manipulation; it is not dependent on the patient being in any particular physical condition or position; and it can be administered in any medical environment.
- Healing sessions support conventional healthcare by reducing fear of treatment or surgery and by alleviating distressing side effects.
- The majority of the population is in favour of having complementary therapies made available on the NHS; and patients are likely to accept healing if offered within an NHS setting.
- Any therapy provided by the NHS must first be approved by NICE. All the research within this book would support an application to NICE.

Promotion of Healing

- More individuals are likely to seek healing if they know that it exists, are aware of the potential benefits and realize that it is natural and normal.
- The media needs to be provided with case studies to report on.
- Individuals who have benefited from healing need to talk openly with others about their experience, including via social media.
- Doctors and other medical professionals need to hear directly from their patients regarding how healing has helped them.

11

Self-Healing

I believe that a significant proportion of the benefit seen from a healing session is due to self-healing; a healer simply helps the recipient to reach the inner state of equilibrium that allows healing to occur. But if seeing a healer is not an option, there is still a great deal that we can do for ourselves quietly at home.

Reading any book about healing or spiritual awareness is likely to be relaxing and uplifting, a state of being that naturally leads to self-healing. Many of these books open the mind to esoteric knowledge, along with practical methods of gaining peace of mind and physical health.

Indeed, people who are sensitive to subtle energies have commented that they notice waves of healing washing over them whenever reading my book. This was my positive intention from the outset, and it is heartening to receive this unsolicited confirmation.

With today's technology, any information is easy to find and available in any chosen medium. YouTube, for instance, offers an Aladdin's cave of free videos that give spiritual guidance, meditations and healing.

A shining example is Esther Hicks,[137] whose discourses cover an incredible depth of knowledge across a vast range of spiritual themes. Despite dealing with serious human issues and deep spiritual truths, her talks are vibrant, engaging and full of humour. She introduces the listener to magnificent concepts and ideas that are both mind-opening and life-enhancing.

Her teachings – collectively referred to as The Law of Attraction – have spawned thousands of books and films on the subject. The core message is that we need to love ourselves unconditionally, and this wholesome and creative energy then shines out into our relationships and into our future.

Esther's ideas are mirrored in Rhonda Byrne's book *The Secret*, which is a delicious pleasure to read. Beautifully designed, each page delivers a bite-sized life lesson. An impressive line-up of leading motivational speakers and teachers add their insights to the respective topics.

The underlying message, though, is not new. Some of the teachers quoted in Rhonda's book date from the 1800s.

Ian Lawton's well-researched book *The Power of You* trawls historical writings as well as modern sources. He presents a wealth of evidence to show that we have been provided with these same lessons for generations. He delivers a flow of enriching gems that serve as reminders for us to keep focused on what matters.

The bottom line of everything taught, in essence, is to be happy.

So many things can separate us from feeling genuinely happy, and most of those only exist in our heads. All worries are about what has happened in the past, or what might happen in the future. But the past is gone, and the imagined future never arrives. We cannot "be alive" in the past, and we cannot "be living" in the future. Only this moment now has life. Choosing to make every "now" moment a positive one is the only logical choice.

Some people have complained to me that they cannot think positively because they have always been a worrier. But if they are not in charge of their own thoughts, then who is?

Negative thinking can be a habit, and noticing an unhelpful thought is a step forward. First, we need to congratulate ourselves for noticing it. There is nothing to be gained from beating ourselves up for having yet another negative thought. That would be a negative thought about the negative thought we just had! Whatever the subject matter, we can think of a collection of positive statements about the same thing. For instance, we might be worried about getting to an appointment on time. Instead, we can feel appreciative that we have the means to get to it – a car, a bus, our legs, money, clothes. We can joyfully imagine that the route is being cleared for us, so we arrive safely and on time. If something does happen to block our path, then we can imagine that this has saved us from an accident further along. We may as well uplift ourselves in these ways because whatever actually happens, will happen anyway. It is only our emotional response to it that really matters.

If the negative thought was about a particular person, then try dwelling upon all the positive points about that same individual. When we hold a grudge, it is only our own selves that suffer. The person who is the target of our angst probably goes gaily about their daily life oblivious to our poisoned arrows. Reeling off all the good points about that person, we may find that we have focused on the 2 per cent that we were unhappy about. If we focus on the 98 per cent instead, our brighter thoughts will overwhelm the measly 2 per cent and we can regain our inner equilibrium.

Forgiving ourselves is as important as forgiving others. We can list our own good points and revel in being better people than we first thought ourselves to be.

A golden nugget of knowledge in Eckhart Tolle's book *A New Earth* is that any thought or feeling that is less than joyful is the ego at work. Simply by noticing a negative thought weakens the ego. The ego is rooted in the left brain, the part of our mind that focuses on our survival and is on the lookout for dangers, real or imagined. Weakening the fears within it leaves more space for the right brain's activity to be noticed, which encompasses the joy of life, loving and being loved, feeling abundant and creative.

The left brain would say that we are human beings having a spiritual experience. The right brain would say that we are spiritual beings having a human experience. The latter is the truth.

Unhelpful thinking devours energy and is insatiable. It takes an inordinate amount of effort to feel stressed. The more we dissolve the ideas that cause the stress, the more energy we have available to live life vibrantly, generating enriching ideas that naturally lead to better physical health.

Keeping abreast of the news has the opposite effect, because the stories tend to be a stream of murder and mayhem. Hardly any good news is reported. Drama sells, and we love it – so long as that drama is about someone else. Reducing our exposure to the news is better for our health and well-being. We do need to know what is happening in our world, and we must admire the journalists who bring contentious issues into the limelight so they can be dealt with. But we do not need to be addicted to the news. What is the point in knowing about disturbing events that we can do nothing about? Or, worse, knowing we can do something but not doing it? If there is a particular issue that we can do something constructive about, then let us take whatever action is possible and then leave it.

There are "good news" newspapers to be found on the internet, such as The Good News Network.[138] Any reading material, radio programmes, films or TV shows that make us laugh or feel cosy inside have an uplifting and therefore physically beneficial impact.

Motivating ourselves to focus on self-healing is key. A severe condition will grip all of our attention, and spur us into action. Lesser issues are easy to ignore because they do not take over our every living moment. But a small problem is like a tap on the shoulder to deal with an underlying cause, and if we ignore that small problem, another larger tap on the shoulder may arrive. Nipping an issue in the bud is by far the best route. All of us have at least several minor problems, either physical or emotional. Nobody is perfect.

My motivation for combating a minor ailment or emotional issue is to think of our son. According to many sources, we are all connected, and most especially with those we hold dear. It follows, then, that if I have a problem it will affect him – either now or in the future – and I would do anything to avoid that. Thinking this way propels me into self-healing activities. Think of someone you love whose health and well-being means so much to you that you are determined to take positive action without delay.

There was a particular time when I worried about our son's immediate future so much that I made myself physically ill for several days. As soon as I could tolerate getting out of bed, a wonderful healer visited to give me healing. The moment he began, I had the clearest vision of me whacking our son about the legs with a heavy bamboo stick. It represented the awful effect of my worrisome thoughts, knocking our son's legs from under him. I resolved to transform my thoughts immediately to those that celebrated every positive aspect of the same situation – and I found there were many. I had a remarkable recovery, and our son's immediate future was successful and exciting.

Finding extra time in our day to relax or meditate can be a challenge, so making use of sleep time extends our opportunities. Last thing at night, lying in bed, listen to the *Sleep Easy & Be Well* CD. Deep and nourishing sleep alone aids healing, but the statements and ideas on the CD lull the subconscious into dissolving fears and stress.

First thing in the morning, when you are still in bed, put your headphones back on and listen to a different recording, one that sets positive intentions for a bright new day. If you like the idea of receiving healing from angels, then Melanie Beckler offers a beautiful range of free YouTube meditations.

If you prefer something more down to earth, Jason Stephenson would be an excellent choice.

For those who favour healing music, rather than spoken word, there are some wonderful options. One of my favourites is Jayson Stilwell, who is a gifted overtone singer. Jayson spent time with throat singers in Tuva (a republic between Siberia and Mongolia) to develop his talent. His unworldly album *Onearth* is a creation entirely of his own voice, no instruments.

Tim Wheater's mesmerizing instrumental music has triggered the most profound effects within me. His album *Golden Light* was particularly created for healing.[139]

Gregorian chant, gongs, singing bowls, drumming, whalesong and chanting are examples of sounds associated with healing. Nature sounds, synthesised harmonies and many more amazing soundscapes can be easily found on the internet, where you can discover and gather your own list of favourites. They can be played in the background to infuse your day, or used as a focused meditation.

Weaving healing ideas into the fabric of our day is another time-saver. Here are some examples.

The words "no" and "not" are quite obviously negative, and they have a subtly downbeat effect upon us. Instead, we can say what we do want, not what we do not want. For instance, teachers are taught to tell children to "Walk!" down the corridor. If they say "Do not run!" children only hear the word "run". Another example is that some people believe that eating organic food will help ward off cancer, but this attitude gives mind space to the destructive thought of cancer. Thinking of positive reasons for eating organic food fills the mind with wholesome beliefs, and the notion of a bright and healthy future.

Weave the word "yes" into your thoughts and language. The word has a freeing and healing quality. Sit for a moment, eyes closed, and thoroughly relax. Now mentally or verbally repeat the word "no" over and over, and note any changes in the body. Then let go of the word "no" and resume your restful state. Now mentally or verbally repeat the word "yes" and note any differences. Some people feel tension accompanying the word "no", while others have a dark colour appear in their mind's eye; or perhaps one hand slightly twitches. When the word "yes" is introduced, some people sense their muscles relax, or a bright colour, or the other hand twitches. If you can master this technique, you can use your body as a diviner to answer questions that need a yes or no response.

Our mind believes everything we say, so we need to watch our words. If we say "my pen" or "my body" we are stating that it belongs to us. Being possessive creatures, we do not like parting with anything that belongs to us. So, rather than saying "my cancer" or "my arthritis" we can separate it from ourselves by saying "the cancer" or "the arthritis". Creating a gap between it and us makes it a separate thing; it no longer belongs to us and is free to leave.

If we say, "I always make mistakes" then we always will. If we say, "I never win raffles" then we never will. What we say now scatters seeds of that potential into our future moments. We can put these same limiting statements safely into the past by saying, "I have made a lot of mistakes", "I have never won a raffle". We are still speaking the truth, but the door is left open for brighter possibilities in the future.

If we say, "I am hopeless at maths" our mind hears, "I am hopeless". Not only will we continue to be hopeless at maths, but it strengthens the sense of hopelessness, which can spread its demoralizing odour into other areas of our life. On every occasion, the phrase "I am" needs to be followed by a positive adjective. Practice some and play with the idea.

The same applies to fearfulness. If one particular fear is allowed to strengthen, then the sensation of fear can spread into other aspects. Fear limits the scope of our life experience, affects our relationships and undermines our confidence.

The energy of fear is the same as exhilaration; only our perception makes them feel so different. When fear rises, try thinking, "This is exhilarating! Gosh, this is exhilarating!" and notice the difference. This worked for me when I gave a talk at the Houses of Parliament.

The phrase "Feel the fear and do it anyway" is excellent advice. When the sensation of fear rises, relax all the muscles, open the mouth and throat and breathe deeply, making no sound. This technique comes from Bert Hellinger,[140] a psychotherapist who began developing his remarkably successful methods in 1987. Try sitting comfortably, bringing to mind a fear and practising this technique.

Addictions are rooted in negative emotions that are so powerful that they override logic. For instance, there is no argument to the logical facts that smoking is terrible for health and finances. The same logical conclusion applies to overeating, alcoholism and drug-taking. Yet people knowingly continue down these paths of self-destruction. What else could be making that decision, other than emotion? An equal and opposite emotion is needed to regain balance. When I gave up smoking, I found a powerful reason why smoking could not be allowed a place in my life, now or ever. I had learned that children of smoker parents are more likely to become smokers themselves. Armed with invincible resolve to pull this addiction out by the roots, I booked a hypnosis session, which worked immediately and permanently.

Another outward sign of inner struggle is the condition of our home. Disarray in our house can be a reflection of the work that needs to be done within. When we clean out cupboards and drawers, and put our belongings into orderly fashion, similar work is automatically occurring within ourselves. If your house is chaotic and seems overwhelming, identify just one small cupboard to clean and tidy, and give yourself a time limit to complete the task. You could put an appointment in your diary and imagine that you are a hired hand, booked to do the work. While doing this job, think of no other work that needs doing. Appreciate the cupboard and everything in it. Do whatever makes the task seem lighter. Once done, stand back and admire your achievement, congratulate yourself, give yourself a healthy treat, and then make an appointment for a slightly larger project. Revisit your cupboard often and revel in its new beauty.

Play relaxing music in the background while you work. People usually find nature sounds soothing, such as birdsong, jungle noises or lapping waves. A calming room scent adds to the mix. Or you might prefer to play your favourite dance music to give you pep.

Gaze around each room of your home and remove any items that do not please you. Anything that makes you smile needs to be in prime position so you see it often. Think about changing the decor to introduce colours that uplift, or feel nurturing and homely. Perhaps add mirrors to bring in more light.

Decluttering is cathartic, and everything you decide to part with can be sold, donated to charity, or given to friends. Be ruthless and let someone else enjoy your pre-loved cast-offs.

Once the house is finished, get into the garden and work your magic there. Tiny tasks first, if that suits you better. Aim for minimum effort for maximum impact, at least to start with.

Inspect your wardrobe and cast out anything that does not suit you, does not fit properly or is outdated. Discard anything you consider suitable only for wearing around the house. Resolve to wear the items you have kept for special occasions as often as possible. Have a look at the colour of your clothes and see if they make you feel uplifted. If not, experiment with brighter hues and see if they make you feel different.

Make time to do things that you enjoy. Be brave and join clubs and classes, go to workshops, immerse yourself in whatever makes you feel more alive. A middle-aged friend spent every evening watching television with her husband because he did not want to go out. Their friends were forever trying to entice her to leave him behind and go out with them to lively bars and dances. She eventually did so, and enjoyed herself so much she started going several times a week. Her husband was glum about being left alone, so eventually he joined them; and he was a changed man! They had so much fun together that they felt years younger.

If you would love to go dancing or rock climbing but your body cannot, then spend time vividly imagining doing that activity. Your body does not know the difference between actually doing and just imagining. By visualizing the activity in your mind, as though it really is happening, your body pumps out the positive hormones and chemicals that accompany joy, which in turn support health.

Learn to enjoy the things you cannot avoid. When washing up, for instance, be grateful that you had food on the table. Be glad that you have family and friends to enjoy meals with. Appreciate that you have clean water coming out of the tap. Give thanks that you have a house to eat in. Feel blessed for the abundance of even the smallest things.

Walk in nature and marvel at its complexity and beauty. Soak it up. Breathe it in. Thoroughly enjoy.

These ideas only touch on the many and varied ways in which we can assist our own healing. If the task seems too daunting, book a series of healing sessions. Over the weeks, you will most likely find yourself achieving these goals naturally and effortlessly.

You might also like to consider downloading "A Gift from Your Self to Yourself" from my website: www.healinginahospital.uk. This self-healing workshop will aid your progress. A seasoned healer watched a section of it and counted 20 beneficial ideas that were either new to her or served as uplifting reminders.'

As previously discussed, I had suffered with psoriasis since my teens, and it was my quest for a cure that led me to spiritual healing. Thanks to a combination of spiritual healing and the above enriching practices, this – medically incurable – condition has now faded away and disappeared.

Key Points

- Self-help techniques can trigger and/or support the healing process.
- Basic healer training is valuable for self-healing and for treating loved ones.
- Being equipped to help ourselves or others is empowering.
- Read books and watch videos that give self-healing guidance or spiritual upliftment.
- Listen to a guided healing meditation last thing at night and first thing in the morning.
- Read books or watch programmes and films that make you laugh.
- Discover activities that make your heart sing.
- Limit the amount of time you spend with negative people.
- Use positive words after "I am ..." and "my ...".
- Keep your mind focused on the positive elements of this moment now.
- Appreciate everything about your body, your life and your environment.
- Surround yourself with beauty in your home.
- Spend time in nature.
- Live each day as though it is your last.

APPENDIX

Comments Made by
Medical Professionals

The following comments were made by delegates at the Nursing in Practice exhibition described on page 35.

When reading the following statements, it should be borne in mind that these people, mostly nurses, were at a busy conference with a tight schedule. As a result, their healing sessions were shorter than usual, the environment was noisy and there was no privacy. They were not unwell and they did not seek healing. Indeed, most were previously unaware of spiritual healing and were sceptical that it could be beneficial. However, they were intrigued enough to sample a session, and the following is a selection of their observations.

"Excellent. Felt warmth, then tension in my neck released."

"A most exhilarating experience. Felt wonderful and so relaxed."

"Beautiful colours moving around. Very therapeutic."

"A very pleasant experience. Felt some of my emotions coming to the surface."

"Absolutely fascinating. I am really surprised how I felt afterwards and will definitely be looking this up on the web."

"Amazing. My pain has gone."

"I felt as though all my troubles were leaving my body and all happy things entering."

"I was sceptical and didn't want to have a session but my friend recommended it and I'm glad I did. The experience was definitely calming and relaxing. Instantly, my knee felt better."

"I felt so relaxed it was unreal. It's like all negative energy left my body."

"My bad arm and neck felt pins and needles."

"I was sceptical but found it relaxing."

"Strange calming sensations in fingers."

"Left me with a tingling sensation all over. Feel very calm and relaxed."

"I went to a lovely place, unaware of my surroundings."

"Warm, relaxing, tilting feeling. Very peaceful."

"Had a particularly bad night with pain and stress. Much calmer in mind and body now. Ready for the day."

"What a lovely, peaceful time. I feel so much better."

"Excellent way to escape the rat race. Totally relaxing."

"Made my headache disappear."

"Very soothing. Felt electrical or spiritual current all over the body."

"I am hoping that this feeling lasts forever."

"Lovely feeling of being here but not here."

"Very relaxing and a feeling of being by the sea alone."

"Very relaxing. I felt bad energies running out of my body."

"Very calming. I feel chilled out and a feeling of lightness."

"Tingly head; warm right hand. Really enjoyed it."

"Felt relaxed and sleepy, even with all the noise around."

"Very relaxing. Felt light-headed immediately afterwards and then re-energized."

"Reduced tension in shoulders. Very relaxing and calming."

"Feel more relaxed. Felt a movement of energy in my knee."

"I feel strange but in a good way."

"Have not experienced this before but would highly recommend it. Have suffered from a headache all morning. It has gone now."

"Very positive experience. Feel very relaxed. Tingling feeling in legs."

"Really felt tingling at areas where healer's hands were. Felt neck relax and pain relieved."

"Very exciting."

"Amazing experience. Want to find out more."

"I cannot really believe how I felt. It was like a magnet that was pulling my negative energy. I was fully relaxed and will never forget the experience."

"Has eased my painful lower back area."

"Very relaxing. Feeling of internal 'denseness'. Very interesting."

"At the beginning I felt as though pins and needles were travelling through my body. Also, I could feel warm spots on certain points of my joints. Relaxing."

"The most relaxing few minutes in a long time. Felt a little like an Aero bar – bubbly."

"Session was short but effective. Sent my hands very tingly. Felt very relaxed."

"Really felt rays on my head and tummy."

"Could feel where the healer was as areas of my body became hot. Felt tired but rejuvenated at the same time."

"Surprisingly relaxing. Will recommend."

"Good experience. Definitely felt the problem area being healed."

"Love, calmness and a feeling of pureness."

"Could feel the tension/heat through my shoulders and top of head. Thank you."

"An excellent way to relieve stress. Feel energized and relaxed."

"Felt tingling and engulfed in light."

"Excellent. Felt the stress leaving my arms in particular."

"That was amazing. The energy that flows afterwards is wonderful."

"Relaxing but strange. The energy felt very strong and at one stage a little uncomfortable, though not painful."

"Best part of the day! The anxiety I came with has gone."

"Absolutely lovely. I want to learn how to do it."

"Interesting departure from my normal logical thinking. The world is full of mysteries and this made me tingle and relax. Will explore further. Keep up the good work."

"Wonderful. A real uplifter. Would be great for our patients."

"A remarkable healing experience."

"Really good. Felt really light and floaty. My foot stopped itching – it had itched all day until now."

"Very interesting. A cynic now believes!"

"Very calming and relaxing. Felt heat throughout body. Will definitely recommend."

"Absolutely lovely. Relaxing. Beautiful colours. Floating."

"What a very happy, enriching experience."

"Thank you so much for giving me so much peace in this busy life of ours. It has been a truly special experience. "

"Extremely interesting experience. I would definitely recommend this to my friends and patients."

"Brilliant. I didn't think it would work but it did. I was really impressed."

"Excellent! Felt like I was floating "

"Excellent. Felt lovely and the pain in my right foot went away. I would recommend it to anyone."

* * *

Angie Buxton-King was employed as a spiritual healer at a children's cancer unit at University London College Hospital. The foreword to her book *The NHS Healer* was penned by Stephen Rowley, Senior Matron, and is reproduced here with Angie's permission:

"University College London Hospital's haematology unit treats patients with leukaemia and other life-threatening diseases. These treatments are highly intensive and carry risks of morbidity and mortality in themselves ... Introducing a spiritual healer into this pressure cooker environment was considered a risk ... We have seen patients with uncontrolled pain find more relief from healing than intramuscular opiates; we have seen patients in psychological

states of utter desperation find, in healing, huge comfort and coping abilities; we have seen patients report significant reductions in chemotherapy-related side effects; we have seen the positive effect healing can have on the troubled, dying patient. Working in this field is demanding and many staff have felt the need for healing themselves and have found significant benefit from doing so.

Healing is the most popular and well received complementary therapy we provide on the unit."

Frequently Asked Questions

Supporting evidence that underpins the statements made within this section is presented within the main body of the book.

What is spiritual healing?

Spiritual from the Latin "spiritus", means "breath of life".
Healing means "making well".
Healing is experienced by many people as a relaxing method of transforming physical pain, unhelpful thoughts and negative emotions into constructive energy. This upcycling of energy then naturally brings about health, peace of mind and vitality.

When the mind experiences a deeply blissful state, the body returns to "biological homeostasis", which is its natural state of balance and self-repair.[141] The deep sense of peace that many people experience during a healing session, coupled with the sensations they report, suggests that they experience this state.

The term "spiritual healing" leads some people to assume that it must be connected to a religion, but this is not the case. Healers do usually believe in a "great creator" or a "universal mind" but not necessarily within an orthodox religious context.

Regarding the possibility of a higher power, one of the world's leading scientists was prompted by a patient to consider the notion. Dr Francis Collins, head of the world-renowned Human Genome Project, explains in his book *The Language of God* how the sciences convinced him to abandon his atheist beliefs.[142]

To avoid being linked with religion, there are healers who prefer to use the term "energy healing" instead. However, this can be misleading because some patients understand it to mean that healing will only help their energy levels, not their physical problems or emotional state.

A number of healers do belong to traditional religions but, whatever their creed, those who are members of a reputable organization will not mention their own beliefs unless the patient specifically asks. Some methods of healing have a long history in their country of origin e.g. spiritual healing in the UK, and reiki in Japan. Others have been developed relatively recently, such as Therapeutic Touch in the USA.

The life force energy that is utilized in healing is referred to as "prana" in Indian languages and "chi" in Chinese culture.

How can healing help someone?

Healing is holistic, meaning that it addresses the person as a whole, not just the symptoms. The word "holistic" is derived from the word "whole".

People often find that healing helps no matter what the problem is. Physical problems, pain, mental anguish and emotional turmoil have all been reported as being alleviated to some degree. Occasionally, recovery has been remarkable by any standards, and several examples of that are offered in this book.

Any reduction of pain, fear, stress and worry is of benefit to our quality of life. A wealth of supporting research indicates that a reduction in these negative feelings improves our physical health and well-being.

What if I am already seeing my doctor?

Healing is complementary to any other treatment, medical or otherwise. It works well used alongside conventional medicine, procedures and surgery. Medical attention should always be sought for a health issue that is causing concern.

How does it work?

There are many ideas and theories, but probably nobody truly knows how healing works. Even people who passionately espouse a convincing hypothesis cannot prove that what they are describing is true.

Training courses often teach that energy flows through the healer into the patient, like water, and that the healer turns the flow on and off, like a tap. In the same way as the pipe gets wet bringing water to the tap, the healer benefits from the positive energy passing through him.

An alternative explanation is that the healer generates a blissful vibration that stimulates the patient's energy into a similar state. This is called entrainment. A physical example of entrainment is where a tuning fork is struck and its sound waves activate an identical tuning fork nearby. Even though the second fork has not been touched, it picks up the vibration from the air and sounds its note. A less known fact is that heart cells in a Petri dish will start beating in rhythm even if they are not touching each other.[143] Similarly, when the healer attunes to the healing vibration, the patient then entrains towards this level. ECGs visibly demonstrate this phenomenon in action. Consequently, I believe that patients can consciously encourage self-healing by surrendering to the process. Healers simply help them to reach that point.

No matter how healing might work, though, the fundamental point is that it does.

Is it just placebo?

The placebo effect is when the recipient's belief in a therapy causes a positive outcome. If someone believes that a pill will help them, it generally does. Placebo is a powerful ally to any form of healing, whether conventional medicine or natural healing. Healthcare professionals and therapists alike would do well to maximize its potential for the benefit of their patients.

It is probably of no importance to the patient whether the positive results of a healing session are due to spiritual energy or to the placebo effect. The evidence is that, at the very least, healing helps unleash the patient's innate and powerful ability to self-heal.

However, healing on animals and plants removes the possibility of the placebo effect because these entities clearly cannot have a belief in the therapy. Yet a range of research shows that healing remains effective for these non-human cases. Even giving healing to human tissue in Petri dishes, under laboratory conditions, registers a positive effect.

Does a patient need to believe in healing for it to work?

No. For example, the two hospital audits described in this book explain that the 267 patients involved did not seek healing and, except for a few, had never contemplated having healing. Some of them strongly believed that healing could not help them, yet it did and, in some cases, remarkably so.

Spiritual healing is often confused with "faith healing", where the patient is told that they must believe in a particular doctrine, deity or ritual for it to work.

As mentioned already, research studies reveal that animals and plants respond to healing, and these serve to demonstrate that belief on the recipient's part is not necessary for healing to be effective.

Babies have no belief system yet they often respond well to healing. One example is a babe in arms who was brought to our voluntary healing centre. She was constantly crying and unable to sleep. No remedy could be found by either her mother or the doctor. After one healing session, the baby slept normally.

Does the healer need to know what the matter is?

No. In the same way that energy from the food we eat naturally goes to where it is most needed, healing energy finds its own way to the core of a problem. As the healer does not need to direct the energy, it is not necessary for the patient to explain what the problem is. This is a relief for people who would be embarrassed to divulge their personal information. They may have a medical problem that embarrasses them, or there may be something in their past or in their behaviour that they are ashamed of.

Also, if a healer knows what the physical problem is, they might concentrate on that particular part and miss the root cause of the issue. For instance, a thumb that has lost its grip can be due to a trapped nerve in the neck, and pain in the lower back can be caused by stress. If the whole body is treated, nothing can be overlooked.

What happens in a healing session?

The patient simply sits or lies down with their eyes closed. There may be soft background music to encourage relaxation. If the person is more comfortable without their coat or shoes, that is fine, but otherwise they remain fully clothed. The healer may then offer a few words of guidance to help the patient unwind further.

If trained by the Healing Trust, the healer takes about 20 minutes to work around the person and complete the session. The healer works with their hands about ten inches (25 cm) away from the body, except for a light touch on the shoulders and feet. The whole of the body is always treated, not just the part that is unwell.

If the healer chooses to work with touch, this is very light and only on the joints of the arms and legs. The healer will always ask permission before using touch of any sort. If the patient agrees to it, I prefer to use touch because the person then knows where I am; and the human touch can also be an added comfort. Some people are not touched by anyone, day after day, and others are only touched by medical professionals or by people who want something. A touch that demands nothing in return can be deeply supportive and reassuring. During a healing session, a patient may feel heat, cold or tingling. They may have involuntary muscle jumps or see colours in their mind's eye. Their eyes may water or they may give a spontaneous deep sigh or two. Sometimes a pain, a feeling of discomfort or an emotion might rise to the surface and then quickly and gently dissipate. Equally, a patient may not sense anything at all. Every response is perfectly normal.

How many sessions are needed?

Just one session has made an astonishing difference to some patients. More typically, a series of five or six weekly sessions brings enough improvements for the patient to start noticing the difference. Some people who make a complete recovery nevertheless choose to continue with sessions to maintain their health and well-being. A man with lifelong mental and emotional problems came to our voluntary healing group every week for many years, saying that it kept him from feeling suicidal. Others simply wish to free themselves of the week's stress and recharge their batteries, just as they might do by going to a gym or a yoga class.

Can healing help someone with a terminal condition?

Yes, but not necessarily to make them live longer. For many people, the dread of dying melts away during a healing session, allowing them to live more contentedly for whatever limited time that they have left. People with a terminal condition are often fearful about how their worsening symptoms will affect them in the future. Others worry about leaving their loved ones behind or parting with their home and possessions. These concerns are often alleviated or brought into perspective as a result of healing.

What is distant healing?

The terms "distant healing", "distance healing" and "absent healing" all refer to the same thing. They mean that the healer is not physically present with the patient, and instead "sends" the healing.

As with prayer, there is no need for the recipient to know that they are being sent healing, and their permission is not required. Numerous groups arrange to send healing; some physically meet together, while others set a weekly time when anyone can add to the collective effort from the comfort of their own home. Healing can be sent to individuals, companies, organizations, governments, to trouble spots and disaster areas around the world, to animals and plants, and to our beleaguered host planet, the Earth.

Do healers "pick up" private information about the patient?

Let us assume, for a moment, that it is possible for personal details to be picked up by a psychic person who is attempting to do so. In every case, accessing private information without permission is wholly unethical. It does not happen as long as the healer has been trained properly and belongs to a reputable organization that has a professional code of conduct. A list of healing organizations appears at the back of this book.

Where is healing available and can it be provided on the National Health Service (UK)?

Healing is available at voluntary healing centres throughout the country, as well as from private practitioners. Doctors can prescribe healing but the NHS might not pay for it. A few surgeries and hospitals have been offering healing at their premises for many years, some by salaried practitioners and others by volunteers. There are also doctors who make rooms available at their surgeries for patients to receive healing, where the patient pays a small fee directly to the healer.

Some religions offer healing; there is no need to belong to their creed to take advantage of this service. Spiritualist churches have always offered healing on a regular basis but some mainstream churches, such as Roman Catholic and Anglican, now offer laying-on of hands. In some churches the healing is delivered only by the priest, while others allow lay people to administer.

Can anyone become a healer?

Yes, everyone has the potential to become a healer. Some people are aware of their natural ability from a young age, while the rest of us have to learn from scratch to develop the skill. Healing is an art, and some people have a natural flair for it, as they might for any other creative pursuit. For instance, some people can cook or sew without effort and others learn languages with ease. The rest of us can manage these activities, but it takes more effort to learn and become proficient. Likewise, with healing everyone has the ability but some need to start with the basics and be determined to progress.

My view is that patients actually heal themselves; the healer simply provides the environment that activates the natural process. Therefore, I believe that those who respond especially well to healing would be particularly ideal candidates for training.

Medical professionals, carers and therapists are likely to be natural healers, having already been drawn to vocations that bring comfort to those in need.

Why train?

Healing is a natural and powerful energy and, like electricity, has simple rules for its safe and effective use. With proper training, a healer cannot become drained as a result of giving healing or be negatively affected in any other way. Indeed, the act of giving healing benefits the healer by virtue of achieving an uplifted state, which in itself accrues health benefits.

People who have a career involving tending to others, or who are caring for a loved one, would especially benefit from learning the basics. Medical professionals, carers and complementary therapists are very often natural healers without realizing it. Looking after the sick and needy can be draining, and learning to regain and maintain the integrity of one's own energies is essential. Also, by adding basic healing knowledge to their skillset, healthcare workers could enhance their patients' experience in the many ways described in this book.

Training to become a healer and putting into practice the philosophies that underpin healing lead to a happier, healthier and more enriched life.

For a list of reputable training organizations, see page 228.

Can people help themselves to heal without proper training?

Yes. This fascinating and empowering area of experiential learning is the subject of many books and workshops. People can be guided towards dissipating long-standing issues, and be introduced to constructive methods of dealing with life's inevitable challenges. Various ideas and resources are offered on page 203 and from page 228 onwards.

What does CAM mean?

Complementary and Alternative Medicine (CAM) includes two different groups. Complementary therapies are those that complement any other form of healthcare and can be used alongside conventional treatment. They do not interfere with the beneficial aspects of medication or surgery.

Spiritual healing falls into this category. Alternative therapies, as the name suggests, are a substitute for conventional medical treatment and purport to provide diagnostic information.

In practice, the term "complementary therapies" is often used to mean both categories, despite the important difference.

What is the difference between reiki and spiritual healing?

Reiki is a Japanese word meaning "spiritual healing" or "universal life energy", and there are a number of different types of reiki. Each healing method is probably slightly different from every other, but the essence is most likely the same. If there is variance in a patient's experience between different styles of healing, this could be due to the healer rather than to the method or modality.

Reiki is widespread because any practitioner who has completed the reiki courses 1, 2 and 3 can teach others without approval or accreditation by a central organization. There are no national standards to be adhered to regarding the course content or the tutor's credentials. Training is therefore abundantly available, and practitioners are easy to find. This ease of access has led to its huge popularity, which has been a tremendous boost for raising public awareness of healing.

Whether using a reiki practitioner or a spiritual healer, patients should ensure that the therapist belongs to a reputable organization. A list is given on page 228.

What is the Healing Trust?

The National Federation of Spiritual Healers (NFSH) was established in 1954, soon after healing became legal in the UK. In recent years, it adopted the working title of "the Healing Trust" to convey its purpose succinctly, with a name that people can easily remember. It has no affiliation with any religion, its members hailing from all faiths and none. Over the decades, erstwhile members have spawned many of the other healing organizations that now exist in the UK and around the world. However, the Healing Trust is probably still the largest healer membership organization. It is the only healing charity to employ salaried staff.

Only trainers accredited by the Healing Trust can provide training, and they teach to a national curriculum. Students are required to become members of the organization before they can advance beyond the initial training course. Becoming a member involves providing personal references and finding qualified healers who are prepared to sponsor the applicant throughout their training. Members are subject to a minimum of two years' training period, final assessment, a professional code of conduct and disciplinary procedures. These standards are designed to give the public confidence that Healing Trust practitioners are respectable and have been trained well.

Experienced practitioners, often volunteers, run support groups for trainee healers throughout the UK and in some other countries. Volunteer members also provide a national network of healing centres to make healing accessible and affordable for members of the public.

The Healing Trust has developed a safe and effective method of giving healing that is delivered in a professional and dignified manner. For insurance purposes, and to comply with prevailing best practice requirements, the healer will ask for certain personal details. This information is treated as strictly confidential.

For ease of reading, NFSH/the Healing Trust is referred to throughout this book simply as the Healing Trust.

How much does a healing session cost?

Financially, voluntary healing centres are very accessible as they usually suggest a minimum donation of a nominal amount, or for those who cannot afford to contribute, nothing at all.

Some private healers use a similar donation arrangement while others charge a professional fee. It is always advised to establish the cost before making a booking.

Resources

Simple Techniques That Support Healing

First of all, find a healer with whom you feel at ease and commit yourself to at least five weekly sessions. If you prefer not to have a healer, listen to a healing meditation every day. The following suggestions will help maximize the potential benefits.

During each healing session:

1. Surrender yourself completely to the healing energies.
2. Imagine breathing in brilliant light with each in-breath.
3. Imagine breathing out worries and concerns with every out-breath.
4. Make your body limp and heavy.
5. Sink into the chair.
6. If emotion rises, open the mouth and throat and breathe deeply, making no sound.
7. Relax any muscles that become tense or uncomfortable.
8. Visualize your whole body as a blaze of light.
9. Imagine every cell feeling loved and appreciated.
10. Every time your mind wanders, bring it back.

Quick Technique to Relieve Pain

Quick and simple does not mean less efficient. This technique, although it takes just a few minutes, has worked time and again, and for some people has been 100 per cent effective. I was as thunderstruck as my patients when this worked for me. The key to success is in commandeering every shred of attention for the task and using vivid imagination.

1. Focus the entirety of your attention onto the core of the pain.
2. Totally relax that part of the body.
3. Imagine that part filled with brilliant golden-white light.
4. Imagine the word "yes" reverberating throughout that part.

5. Repeatedly intensify all of the above.
6. Let no other thought enter your mind.
7. If a different colour light presents itself, or is easier to imagine, focus on that colour and make it the brightest possible.

Sleep Easy & Be Well CD

This spoken word recording helps the listener to relax and drift into deep and nourishing sleep. The background sound, with no beat and no chimes, has been designed to be intensely soothing.

Dr Singh gave a copy of this CD to one of his patients who had not slept since her husband died, two years previously. She reported sleeping well from the first time she listened to it. He also gives copies to prison inmates who often report positive effects.

Another patient had been on sleeping tablets for three years but came straight off them when he started listening to this CD.

A friend listened to this while doing the ironing, to check it out before offering it to her wakeful teenage daughter. Despite not using the CD in the manner intended, my friend found that she was no longer afraid of going to the dentist.

To prepare for a good night's sleep, avoid eating for a few hours beforehand and only have bedtime drinks during that time. Drinks that encourage restful sleep include almond milk, malted milk, valerian tea and chamomile tea. If you sleep on your back, you may find that a pillow under the knees helps take pressure off the lower back. Look forward to going to bed and expect to sleep well. Make arrangements not to be disturbed, switch the telephone off and, for the best effect, use headphones.

All proceeds benefit the Healing Trust's charitable work. A copy can be downloaded from:

Website: *www.healinginahospital.uk*

Find a Healer or Training

Healer Organizations

For protection of the public, all healers belonging to the following organizations are subject to a minimum of two years' training, a professional code of conduct and disciplinary procedures. They are also covered by professional insurance. These organizations are not connected to any religion.

NFSH/The Healing Trust

Website: *www.thehealingtrust.org.uk*
Email: *office@thehealingtrust.org.uk*
Tel : *0044 1604 603247*

The Healing Trust is the oldest and probably the largest healer membership organization in the world, offering:

- Voluntary healing groups throughout the UK.
- Find a Healer service (UK and overseas) and distant healing.
- Training to national standards by accredited tutors throughout the UK as well as in America, Australia, Germany, Ireland, New Zealand, Poland and Portugal.
- Support groups for trainees and healers throughout the UK.

Established in 1954, the National Federation of Spiritual Healers (NFSH) was originally an umbrella organization for disparate healing groups throughout the UK. Its first President was Harry Edwards, a famous healer whose public demonstration at the Royal Albert Hall drew an audience of 6,000 people.

In 1976, the NFSH decided to only accept individuals as members, not groups, so that professional elements like training standards could be introduced. Many groups preferred to remain as they were, so they set up a separate umbrella organization for themselves (BAHA). The total number of healers that had originally belonged to NFSH was therefore split between the two organizations.

No longer a federation and no longer only national, the NFSH adopted the working title of "The Healing Trust" in 2009. This name is much easier for people to remember and immediately conveys the purpose of the organization.

NFSH The Healing Trust Training in the USA
Website: *www.nfsh-thehealingtrusttrainingusa.org*
Email: *ksmith727@comcast.net*
Tel: *001(239) 692-9120*

Covering all of America, offering:
- Healer training
- Find a Healer service
- Community healing circles
- Webinars, Meditations

The NFSH (NZ) Inc
Website: *www.nfsh.org.nz*
Email: *bob.jan@xtra.co.nz*
Tel: *0064 7 868 5204*

Covering New Zealand and Australia. Established as a charity in 1996, NFSH (NZ) offers healing and training.

British Alliance of Healing Associations (BAHA)
Website: *www.britishalliancehealingassociations.com*

Established in 1977, BAHA is an umbrella organization for healing groups that meet its standards.

College of Healing
Website: *www.collegeofhealing.org*

Established in 1983 by a group of doctors and healers, the College of Healing was set up as an educational charity. One of its founders, Diane O'Connell, had previously developed healer training courses with colleagues, which they ran in 1975/6. At that time it was generally believed that healing was a gift and could not be taught, but when their pioneering work became known to other healing organizations, they followed suit. Diane continues to be at the forefront of training standards in the UK.

Confederation of Healing Organisations (CHO)

Website: *www.the-cho.org.uk*
Email: *admin @the-cho.org.uk*
Tel: *0044 300 302 0021*

The CHO is an umbrella organization for healing groups that meet its standards. It was created in 1982 by Denis Haviland, who was a prominent industrialist. When he retired due to ill health and arthritis, he was persuaded to receive healing from the wife of a major general. He was soon walking without sticks and, as a result, was inspired to make healing more available and accepted. He formed the CHO with a number of founding organizations, with the aim that healing be made available throughout the NHS.

Harry Edwards Healing Sanctuary

Website: *www.harryedwardshealingsanctuary.org.uk*
Email: *info@burrowslea.org.uk*
Tel: *0044 1483 202054*

Burrows Lea was originally the private home of Harry Edwards, a successful businessman and famous healer. He converted part of the property into a healing sanctuary that continues to offer healing and training.

Healing in America

Website: *www.healinginamerica.com*
Email: *info@healinginamerica.com*
Tel: *001 (805) 640-0211*

Originally linked to the Healing Trust, Healing in America continues its work with the same ethos and values. Their workshops are approved by the American Holistic Nurses Association.

Therapeutic Touch International Association

Website: *www.therapeutictouch.org*
Email: *info@therapeutictouch.org*
Tel: *001 (518) 325 1185*

Originally set up by nurses in America, TT is now also established in many other countries.

UK Healers

Website: *www.ukhealers.info*
Email: *admin@ukhealers.info*

UK Healers is an umbrella organization for healer membership organizations that meet its standards. It is the largest voluntary, professional-standards-setting, accrediting body for the training and practice of spiritual healing.

Reiki Organizations

The Reiki Council

Website: *www.reikicouncil.org.uk*
Email: *info@reikicouncil.org.uk*

The Reiki Council is an umbrella organization for reiki groups that meet its requirements. Its website states that the Council cannot take any liability for reiki practitioners sourced via its member associations.

UK Reiki Federation

Website: *www.reikifed.co.uk*
Email: *enquiry@reikifed.co.uk*

The UK Reiki Federation is a member of the Reiki Council and is one of the largest reiki organizations in the UK. Its website states that it promotes best practice within the field of reiki and stipulates a minimum training period of nine months.

The International Center for Reiki Training

Website: *www.reiki.org*
Email: *center@reiki.org*
Tel: *001 (248) 948 8112*

An American not-for-profit organization, ICRT offers training and Find a Practitioner.

Australian Reiki Connection

Website: *www.australianreikiconnection.com.au*
Tel: *0061 439 366 185*

Established in 1997, ARC is a not-for-profit organization offering training, distant healing and Find a Practitioner.

Reiki Australia

Website: *www.reikiaustralia.wildapricot.org*

A not-for-profit organization offering training and Find a Practitioner

Healing Offered by Religions

Although healing need not be connected to a religion, some readers may wish to consider this option.

Spiritualists National Union (SNU)

Stansted Hall, Stansted, Essex, CM24 8UD
Website: *www.snu.org.uk*
Tel: *0044 1279 816363*

The SNU has always had a strong tradition of healing. It has excellent standards of training, with a minimum period of two years. Healing is usually offered every week at hundreds of its churches around the world. People of any religion or none are welcomed.

Christian Science

Website: *www.christianscience.com*

Established in America in the 1800s, Christian Science began life as a result of a remarkable spiritual healing. Their churches around the world continue to include healing as an intrinsic aspect of their work. Traditionally, their teachings eschewed medical care, but this has now been overturned. Always seek medical care for a medical condition.

Other Churches

Healing is becoming more available at different Christian denominations, even the orthodox ones.

Other Religions

I could find no information to suggest that healing is offered to the public by any other religion.

Healing Research Sources

The Research Council for Complementary Medicine (RCCM)

Address: *c/o John Hughes Ph.D., Royal London Hospital for Integrated Medicine, 60 Great Ormond St, London WC1N 3HR*
Website: *www.rccm.org.uk*
Email: *info@rccm.org.uk*

RCCM was founded in 1983. Its vision is to promote research that will widen the availability of safe and effective complementary medicine.

Wholistic Healing Research

Website: *www.wholistichealingresesarch.com*

Dr Daniel J. Benor has devoted decades of his life to amassing a wealth of research evidence concerning healing. This is presented on his website and also in his books, particularly *Healing Research Volumes I–IV.*

Institute of Noetic Sciences

Website: *www.noetic.org*

Since 1973, IONS has been at the forefront of the scientific investigation of consciousness and its role in our lives. They explore the interconnection between personal, inner space and the "outer space" of our shared reality.

Council for Healing

Website: *www.councilforhealing.org*

The CfH conducts research and provides expert consultation in design and methodology. They also promote awareness of existing research.

Healing in Medical Settings

The Sam Buxton Sunflower Healing Trust

Website: *www.cancertherapies.org.uk*

In 2006, Angie Buxton-King and her husband set up a charity in memory of her young son, who had died of cancer. Since then, it has financed the first two years' salary of over 35 healers working in different NHS hospitals and hospices around the UK. The salary commitment for the majority of these healers has then been taken over by the recruiting NHS centre.

Doctor Healer Network

Website: *www.doctorhealer.org*

The DHN encourages the acceptance and use of integrated medicine, incorporating healing as a major component. It offers information, advice, and a discussion forum for healthcare professionals who wish to become involved in healing. It aims to promote understanding and awareness of healing as a recognized and viable form of complementary therapy and to form collaborative links with medical and healthcare professionals and researchers. Members of the DHN include medical staff, academics as well as complementary therapists who work alongside medical professionals. Approximately 25 per cent of the membership comprises doctors.

Abbreviations

CAM	Complementary and Alternative Medicine
CHO	Confederation of Healing Organisations
ECG	Electrocardiogram
EDA	Electrodermal Activity
EEG	Electroencephalograph (scanner)
FMRI	Functional Magnetic Resonance Imaging (scanner)
FRCGP	Fellow of the Royal College of General Practitioners
GP	General Practitioner – UK term for a family doctor in the community
H-B	Harvey Bradshaw Questionnaire
HIV	Human Immunodeficiency Virus
IBD	Inflammatory Bowel Disease
IBDQ	Inflammatory Bowel Disease Quality-of-Life Questionnaire
IBS	Irritable Bowel Syndrome
IBS-QOL	Irritable Bowel Syndrome Quality-of-Life Questionnaire
ITT	Intention To Treat - all patients, whether or not they received all five healing sessions
LVO	Royal Victorian Order – a British honour
MBS	Mind, Body, Soul/Spirit
MND	Motor Neurone Disease
MRI	Magnetic Resonance Imaging (scanner)
MS	Multiple Sclerosis
MYMOP	Measure Yourself Medical Outcome Profile
NFSH	National Federation of Spiritual Healers (aka The Healing Trust)
NHS	National Health Service (UK)
NICE	National Institute for Health and Care Excellence (UK)
OBE	Order of the British Empire – a British honour
PCT	Primary Care Trust (UK)
PEFR	Peak Expiratory Flow Rate
PP	Per Protocol – only patients who received all five healing sessions
QOL	Quality of Life
RCT	Randomized Controlled Trial
REM	Rapid Eye Movement
SATS	Standard Assessment Tests National curriculum tests (UK)
SCCAI	Simple Clinical Colitis Activity Index Questionnaire
TT	Therapeutic Touch
UC	Ulcerative Colitis

List of Figures

Notes

1. Pesek, T., L. Helton, and M. Nair. "Healing Across Cultures: Learning From Traditions." *EcoHealth* 3 (2006).

2. The Encyclopedia of Earth, Biological Homeostasis, http://www.eoearth.org/view/article/150655

3. Cleveland Clinic, Guided Imagery & Heart Surgery, http://my.cleveland clinic.org/services/heart/prevention/emotional-health/stress-relaxation/guided-imagery-heart-surgery

4. Malmivuo, J., and R. Plonsey. *Bioelectromagnetism: Principles and Applications of Bioelectric and Biomagnetic Fields.* Oxford University Press, 1995.

5. Song, M-Y., M. John, and A. S. Dobs. "Clinicians, Attitudes and Usage of Complementary and Alternative Integrative Medicine." *The Journal of Alternative and Complementary Medicine* 13 (2007); Brown, J. et al. "Complementary and alternative therapies: survey of knowledge and attitudes of health professionals at a tertiary pediatric/women's care facility." *Complementary Therapies in Clinical Practice* 13 (2007); Lorenca, A., M. Blairb, and N. Robinson. "Personal and professional influences on practitioners, attitudes to traditional and complementary approaches to health in the UK." *Journal of Traditional Chinese Medical Sciences* 1 (2014).

6. www.ruthkaye.net

7. www.nhs.uk/conditions/stress-anxiety-depression/mindfulness

8. science.nasa.gov/astrophysics/focus-areas/what-is-dark-energy

9. www.anitamoorjani.com

10. www.dannion.com

11. www.deniselinn.com

12. www.healer.ch

13. www.theinnersourcestore.com

14. www.thework.com

15. www.eckharttolle.com

16. Cousins, N. *Anatomy of an Illness; as perceived by the patient.* W. W. Norton & Co Inc, 2005.

17. www.louisehay.com

18. Institute of Noetic Sciences, Spontaneous Remission Bibliography Project http://www.noetic.org/research/projects/spontaneous-remission

19. Mayo, E. *Hawthorne and the Western Electric Company, The Social Problems of an Industrial Civilisation.* Routledge, 1949.

20. www.sleepcouncil.org.uk

21. Endo, T., C. Roth, H. P. Landolt, and E. Werth. "Selective REM sleep deprivation in humans: Effects on sleep and sleep EEG." *The American Journal of Physiology* 274 (1998).

22. Carey, J. *The Faber Book of Science.* Faber & Faber, London (1995).

23. Denison, B. "Touch the pain away: new research on therapeutic touch and persons with fibromyalgia syndrome." *Holistic Nursing Practice* 18 (2004).

24. www.medicalnewstoday.com/articles/326193. Medically reviewed by Maria Prelipcean, M.D. — Written by Jessica Caporuscio, Pharm.D. on 30 August 2019.

25. www.health.harvard.edu/staying-healthy/understanding-inflammation

26. What is Stress? The Stress Management Society http://www.stress.org.uk /What is stress.aspx

27. Bloom, D. "Instead of detention, these students get meditation." *CNN News.* 2016. edition.cnn.com/2016/11/04/health/meditation-in-schools -baltimore

28. House of Lords – Science & Technology; Sixth Report, Parliament UK – Parliamentary Business; Publications & Records, http://www.parliament .the-stationery-office.co.uk/pa/ld199900/ldselect/ldsctech/123/12301.htm

29. Langmead, L., M. Chitinis, and D. S. Rampton. "Use of complementary therapies by patients with IBD may indicate psychosocial distress." *Inflammatory Bowel Disease* 8 (2002); Kong, S. C., D. P. Hurlstone, C.Y. Pocock et al. "The incidence of self prescribed oral complementary and alternative medicine use by patients with gastrointestinal diseases." *Journal of Clinical Gastroenterology* 39 (2005).

30. Gillespie, E. A., B. W. Gillespie, and M. J. Stevens. "Painful diabetic neuropathy: impact of an alternative approach." *Diabetes Care* 30 (2007).

31. Wilson, S., L. Roberts, A. Roalfe et al. "Prevalence of irritable bowel syndrome: a community survey." *British Journal of General Practice* 54, no. 504 (2004); Akelhurst, R. L. et al. "Health-related quality of life and cost impact of irritable bowel syndrome in a UK primary care setting." *Pharmacoeconomics* 20 (2002); El-Serag, H. B., K. Olden, and D. Bjorkman. "Health-related quality of life among persons with irritable bowel syndrome: a systematic review." *Alimentary Pharmacology & Therapeutics* 16 (2002); Gralnek, I. M., R. D. Hays, A. Kilbourne, B. Naliboff, and E. A. Mayer. "The impact of irritable bowel syndrome on health-related quality of life." *Gastroenterology* 119 (2000); Hungin, A. P., P. J. Whorwell, J. Tack, and F. Mearin. "The prevalence, patterns and impact of irritable bowel syndrome: an international survey of 40,000 subjects." *Aliment Pharmacol Ther* 17 (2003); Feagan, B. G., M. Bala, S. Yan, A. Olson, and S. Hanauer. "Unemployment and disability in patients with moderately to severely active Crohn's disease." *Journal of*

Clinical Gastroenterology 39 (2005); Casellas, F. et al. "Impairment of health-related quality of life in patients with inflammatory bowel disease." *Inflammatory Bowel Disease* 11 (2005).

32. Hungin, A. P., P. J. Whorwell, J. Tack, and F. Mearin. "The prevalence, patterns and impact of irritable bowel syndrome: an international survey of 40,000 subjects." (*Aliment Pharmacol Ther*) 17 (2003); Wilson, S., L. Roberts, A. Roalfe et al. "Prevalence of irritable bowel syndrome: a community survey." *British Journal of General Practice* 54, no. 504 (2004).

33. Rubin, D. T., C. A. Siegel, S. V. Kane et al. "Impact of ulcerative colitis from patients, and physicians, perspectives: Results from the UC: NORMAL survey." *Inflammatory Bowel Disease* 15 (2009).

34. Hahn, B. A. "A review of the Clinical Economics of Irritable Bowel Syndrome." *Annals of Gastroenterology* 15 (2002); Cosnes, J., C. Gower-Rousseau, P. Seksik, and A. Cortot. "Epidermiology and Natural History of Inflammatory Bowel Diseases." *Gastroenterology* 140 (2011).

35. So, P. S., Y. Jiang, and Y. Qin. "Touch therapies for pain relief in adults." *Cochrane Database Systematic Review* 4 (2008).

36. Gordon, A., J. H. Merenstein, F. D'Amico, and D. Hudgens. "The effects of therapeutic touch on patients with osteoarthritis of the knee." *The Journal of Family Practice* 47 (1998); Turner, J.G., A. J. Clark, D. K. Gauthier, and M. Williams. "The effect of therapeutic touch on pain and anxiety in burn patients." *Journal of Advanced Nursing* 28, no. 1 (1998); Denison, B. "Touch the pain away: new research on therapeutic touch and persons with fibromyalgia syndrome." *Holistic Nursing Practice* 18 (2004).

37. So, P. S., Y. Jiang, and Y. Qin. "Touch therapies for pain relief in adults." *Cochrane Database Systematic Review* 4 (2008); Wardell, D. W., and K. F. Weymouth. "Review of Studies of Healing Touch." *Journal of Nursing Scholarship* 36, no. 2 (2004).

38. Barlow, F. V., F. Biley, J. Walker, and G. Lewith. "The experience of spiritual healing for women with breast cancer." *Journal of Complementary Therapies in Medicine* 18 (2010).

39. Rein, G. "A psychokinetic effect of neurotransmitter metabolism: Alterations in the degradative enzyme monoamine oxidase." *Research in Parapsychology*; Scarecrow Press, Metuchen, NJ (1986).

40. Braud, W., Davis, G. and Wood R. "Experiments with Matthew Manning." *Journal of the Society for Psychical Research* Vol 50 (1979).

41. Haraldsson, E. and Thorsteinsson, T. "Psychokinetic effects on yeast: An exploratory experiment." *Research in Parapsychology*, Scarecrow Press, Metuchen, NJ (1973).

42. Tedder, W. H. and Monty, M. L. "Exploration of long-distance PK: A conceptual replication of the influence on a biological system." *Research in Parapsychology* (1980) pp 90–93.

43. Scofield A. M. and Hodges, R. D. "Demonstration of a Healing Effect in the Laboratory using a Simple Plant Model." *Journal of the Society for Psychical Research* Vol 57 (1991).

44. Grad, B. R. "Some biological effects of laying-on of hands: a review of experiments with animals and plants." *Journal of the American Society for Psychical Research* Vol 59 (1965).

45. Wirth, D. P. "Unorthodox healing: the effect of non-contact therapeutic touch on the healing rate of full thickness dermal wounds." journals.sfu.ca /seemj/index.php/seemj/article/view/14

46. Miller, R. N. "Study on the effectiveness of remote mental healing." *Medical Hypotheses* 8 (1982).

47. Keller, E., and V. M. Bzdek. "Effects of therapeutic touch on tension headache pain." *Nursing Research* 35 (1986).

48. Heidt, P. "Effects of therapeutic touch on the anxiety level of hospitalized patients." *Nursing Research* 30 (1981).

49. Quinn, J. F. "An Investigation of the Effect of Therapeutic Touch Without Physical Contact on State Anxiety of Hospitalized Cardiovascular Patients." Unpublished Ph.D. thesis. New York University. Quoted by Benor 1982.

50. Wirth D. P., D. R. Brenlan, R. J. Levine, C. M. Rodriguez. "The effect of complementary healing therapy on postoperative pain after surgical removal of impacted third molar teeth." *Complementary Therapies in Medicine* 1 (1993).

51. Scofield A. M., R. D. Hodges. "Demonstration of a Healing Effect in the Laboratory using a Simple Plant Model." *Journal of the Society for Psychical Research* 57 (1991).

52. Roney-Dougal, S. M., and J. Solfvin. "Field Study of an Enhancement Effect on Lettuce Seeds: A Replication Study." *Journal of Parapsychology* 67 (2003).

53. Hodges R. D. and A. M. Scofield. "Is Spiritual Healing a Valid and Effective Therapy?" *Journal of the Royal Society of Medicine* 88 (1995).

54. Gronowicz, G. A., A. Jhaveri, L. W. Clarke, M. S. Aronow, and T. H. Smith. "Therapeutic Touch Stimulates the Proliferation of Human Cells in Culture." *The Journal of Alternative and Complementary Medicine* 14 (2008); Jhaveri, A., Y. Wang, M. B. McCarthy, and G. A. Gronowicz. "Therapeutic Touch affects proliferation and bone formation of human osteoblasts in vitro." *Journal of Orthopaedic Research* 2008.

55. Abe, K. et al. "Effect of a Japanese energy healing method known as Johrei on viability and proliferation of cultured cancer cells in vitro." *Journal of Alternative and Complementary Medicine* Vol 18 (2012).

56. Gerard, S., B. H. Smith, and J. A. Simpson. "A randomized controlled trial of spiritual healing in restricted neck movement." *Journal of Alternative and Complementary Medicine* 9 (2003).

57. www.wholistichealingresearch.com

58. Astin, J. A., E. Harkness, and E. Ernst. "The efficacy of distant healing: a systematic review of randomised trials." *Annals of Internal Medicine* 132 (2000).

59. Braud, W., and M. Schlitz. "A methodology for the objective study of transpersonal imagery." *Journal of Scientific Exploration* 3 (1989).

60. Warber, S. L., B. W. Gillespie, G. L. M. Kile, D. Gorenflo, and S. F. Bolling. "Meta-analysis of the effects of therapeutic touch on anxiety symptoms." *Focus on Alternative and Complementary Therapies* 5 (2000).

61. Achterberg, J., K. Cooke, T. Richards, L. Standish, L. Kozak, and J. Lake. "Evidence for Correlations Between Distant Intentionality and Brain Function in Recipients: A Functional Magnetic Resonance Imaging Analysis." *The Journal of Alternative and Complementary Medicine* 11 (2005).

62. Arom, K., and B. MacIntyre. "The Effect of Healing Touch on coronary artery bypass surgery patients." Denver: Healing Touch International 6th Annual Conference, 2002.

63. Bunnell, T. "The effect of hands-on healing on enzyme activity." *Research in Complementary Medicine* 3 (1996).

64. Bunnell, T. "The effect of healing on peak expiratory flow rates in asthmatics." *Subtle Energies* 13 (2002).

65. Connor, M. et al. "Extraordinary healing using Resonance Modulation distance energy healing in T6 spinal paraplegia." (Poster session, ISSSEEM meeting) 2004.

66. Creath, K., and G. E. Schwartz. "Measuring effects of music, noise and healing energy using a seed germination bioassay." *The Journal of Alternative and Complementary Medicine* 10 (2004).

67. http://www.mindmirroreeg.com/w/equipment/mm3/unique.htm

68. Radin, D. et al. "Compassionate intention as a therapeutic intervention by partners of cancer patients: effects of distant intention on the patients' autonomic nervous system." *Explore (NY)* Vol 4 (2008).

69. bluebottlelove.com/hew-len-hooponopono

70. Heisenberg, W. *Physics and Beyond.* Harper and Row (1971).

71. Feynman, R. P. *The Character of Physical Law.* Penguin Press Science (1992).

72. Penman, D. Mail Online. http://www.dailymail.co.uk/health/article-408280/Could-spiritual-healing-actually-work.html#ixzz3JhKBM1a7

73. Roe, C. A., C. Sonnex, and E. C. Roxburgh. "Two Meta-Analyses of Non-Contact Healing Studies." *EXPLORE (NY)* Vol 11 (2015).

74. Peters, D. "Why we need a new model for 21st century healthcare." *The Journal of Holistic Healthcare* 2 (2005).

75. Patton, M. *Qualitative evaluation and research method.* Newbury Park, CA: Sage Publications, 1990.

76. Lee, R. T., T. Kingstone, L. Roberts, S. Edwards, A. Soundy, P. R. Shah, M. S. Haque, S. Singh. "A pragmatic randomised controlled trial of healing therapy in a gastroenterology outpatient setting." *European Journal of Integrative Medicine* 9 (2017).

77. Altman, D. G. *Practical Statistics for Medical Research.* Chapman & Hall, 1991.

78. Drossman, D. et al. "Characterization of health related quality of life (HRQOL) for patients with functional bowel disorder (FBD) and its response to treatment." *American Journal of Gastroenterology* 102 (2007).

79. "What is an effect size?" University of Oxford; Centre for Evidence Based Intervention. www.cebi.ox.ac.uk/for-practitioners/what-is-good-evidence/what-is-an-effect-size.html

80. Eisen, S. V., G. Ranganathan, P. Seal, and A. Spiro. "Measuring Clinically Meaningful Change Following Mental Health Treatment." *The Journal of Behavioral Health Services & Research* 34 (2007).

81. Kazis, L. E., J. J. Anderson, and R. F. Meenan. "Effect sizes for interpreting changes in health status." *Medical Care* 27 (1989).

82. Higgins, P. D. R., M. Schwartz, J. Mapili, I. Krokos, J. Leung, and E. M. Zimmermann. "Patient defined dichotomous end points for remission and clinical improvement in ulcerative colitis." *BMJ Gut* 54 (2005).

83. Targan, S. R., F. Shanahan, and L. C. Karp. *Inflammatory Bowel Disease: Translating Basic Science into Clinical Practice.* Wiley-Blackwell, 2011.

84. Crohn's Disease Activity Index. en.wikipedia.org/wiki/Crohn%27s_Disease_Activity_Index

85. Patsopoulos, N. A. "A pragmatic view on pragmatic trials." *Dialogues in Clinical Neuroscience* 13, no. 2 (2011).

86. "IBS and Non-GI Functional Disorders." International Foundation for Gastro Intestinal Disorders. www.aboutibs.org/site/what-is-ibs/other-disorders/non-gi-functional-disorders#table1

87. Parasuraman, A., V. A. Zeithaml, and L. L. Berry. "SERVQUAL: A Multiple-Item Scale for Measuring Consumer Perceptions of Service Quality." *Journal of Retailing* 64 (1988).

88. Soundy, A., R. Lee, T. Kingstone, S. Singh, P. R. Shah, S. Edwards, L. Roberts. "Experiences of healing therapy in patients with irritable bowel syndrome and inflammatory bowel disease." *BioMed Central* 15 (2015).

89. Cohen, L., and L. Manion. *Research Methods in Education.* Routledge, 2000.

90. Beecher, H. K. "The Powerful Placebo." *The Journal of the American Medical Association* 1955.

91. Kienle, G. S. and H. Kiene. "The powerful placebo effect: fact or fiction?" *Journal of Clinical Epidemiology* 50 (1997).

92. Hróbjartsson, A. and P. C. Gøtzsche. "Is the Placebo Powerless? An Analysis of Clinical Trials Comparing Placebo with No Treatment." *The New England Journal of Medicine* 344 (2001).

93. Kaptchuk, T. J., J. M. Kelley, L. A. Conboy et al. "Components of placebo effect: randomised controlled trial in patients with irritable bowel syndrome." *British Medical Journal* 336 (2008).

94. Moseley, J. B. et al. "A Controlled Trial of Arthroscopic Surgery for Osteoarthritis of the Knee." *The New England Journal of Medicine* (2002).

95. Sihvonen R. et al. "Arthroscopic Partial Meniscectomy versus Sham Surgery for a Degenerative Meniscal Tear." *The New England Journal of Medicine* (2013).

96. Wager, T. D., L. Y. Atlas, L. A. Leotti, and J. K. Rilling. "Predicting Individual Differences in Placebo Analgesia: Contributions of Brain Activity during Anticipation and Pain Experience." *The Journal of Neuroscience* 31(2) (2011).

97. hms.harvard.edu/news/placebome

98. *House of Lords – Science & Technology; Sixth Report.* 1999–2000. www.parliament.the-stationery-office.co.uk/pa/ld199900/ldselect /ldsctech/123/12301.htm

99. Lee, R. T., T. Kingstone, L.Roberts, S. Edwards, A. Soundy, P.R. Shah, M. S. Haque, S. Singh. "A pragmatic randomised controlled trial of healing therapy in a gastroenterology outpatient setting." *European Journal of Integrative Medicine* 9 (2017).

100. Soundy, A., R. Lee, T. Kingstone, S. Singh, P. R. Shah, S. Edwards, L. Roberts."Experiences of healing therapy in patients with irritable bowel syndrome and inflammatory bowel disease." *BioMed Central* 15 (2015).

101. Bassi, A., S. Dodd, P. Williamson, and K. Bodger. "Cost of illness of inflammatory bowel disease in the UK: a single centre retrospective study." *Gut* 53, no. 10 (2004).

102. *House of Lords Publications; Lords Hansard; Daily Hansard.* 29 May 2001. www.publications.parliament.uk/pa/ld200001/ldhansrd /vo010329/text/10329-13.htm (accessed May 12 2015). *Parliament UK - Parliamentary Business; Publications & Records.*

103. Baldwin, E. *A Look at CAM.* s406515300.onlinehome.us/lookatcambyl. html.

104. *House of Lords – Science & Technology; Sixth Report.* 1999-2000 www.parliament.the-stationery-office.co.uk/pa/ld199900/ldselect /ldsctech/123/12301.htm

105. Ibid.

106. *House of Lords Publications; Lords Hansard; Daily Hansard.* 29 May 2001. www.publications.parliament.uk/pa/ld200001/ldhansrd/ vo010329/text/10329-13.htm (accessed May 12 2015). *Parliament UK - Parliamentary Business; Publications & Records.*

107. Weze, C., H. L. Leathard, J. Grange, P. Tiplady, and G. Stevens. "Evaluation of healing by gentle touch." *Journal of the Royal Institute of Public Health* 2004.

108. Weze, C., H. L. Leathard, J. Grange, P. Tiplady, and G. Stevens. "Evaluation of healing by gentle touch in 35 clients with cancer." *European Journal of Oncology Nursing* 2003.

109. Weze, C., H. L. Leathard, J. Grange, P. Tiplady, and G. Stevens. "Healing by Gentle Touch Ameliorates Stress and Other Symptoms in People Suffering with Mental Health Disorders or Psychological Stress." *Evidence-Based Complementary and Alternative Medicine* 2006.

110. Shore, A. G. "Long-term effects of energetic healing on symptoms of psychological depression and self-perceived stress." *Alternative Therapies in Health and Medicine* 10, no. 4 (2004).

111. Marta, I. E., S. S. Baldan, A. F. Berton, M. Pavam, and M. J. da Silva. "The effectiveness of therapeutic touch on pain, depression and sleep in patients with chronic pain: clinical trial." *Journal of the Nursing School of the University of Sao Paulo* 44 (2010).

112. Wardell, D. W., and K. F. Weymouth. "Review of Studies of Healing Touch." *Journal of Nursing Scholarship* 36, no. 2 (2004).

113. Dixon, M. "Does healing benefit patients with chronic symptoms? A quasi-controlled trial in general practice." *Journal of the Royal Society of Medicine* Vol 91 (1998). www.ncbi.nlm.nih.gov/pmc/articles/PMC1296636/

114. Brown, C. K. "Is spiritual healing a valid and effective therapy?" *Journal of the Royal Society of Medicine* Vol 88 (1995). www.ncbi.nlm.nih.gov/pmc/articles/PMC1295432/?page=1

115. Cani, P. D., M. Osto, L. Geurts, and A. Everard. "Involvement of gut microbiota in the development of low-grade inflammation and type 2 diabetes associated with obesity." *Gut Microbes* 3 (2012); Frazier, T. H., J. K. DiBaise, and C. J. McClain. "Gut Microbiota, Intestinal Permeability, Obesity-Induced Inflammation, and Liver Injury." *Journal of Parenteral and Enteral Nutrition* 35 (2011); de la Serre, C. B., G. de Lartigue, and H. E. Raybould. "Chronic exposure to low dose bacterial lipopolysaccharide inhibits leptin signaling in vagal afferent neurons." *Physiology & Behavior* 139 (2015).

116. Evrensel, A., and M. E. Ceylan. "The Gut–Brain Axis: The Missing Link in Depression." *Clinical Psychopharmacology and Neuroscience* 13, no. 3 (2015).

117. www.galileocommission.org

118. www.rccm.org.uk

119. www.noetic.org

120. Lazara, S. W. et al. "Meditation experience is associated with increased cortical thickness." *NeuroReport* 16 (2005).

121. Diener, E., and M. Y. Chan. "Happy People Live Longer: Subjective Wellbeing Contributes to Health and Longevity." *Applied Psychology: Health and Wellbeing* 3 (2011).

122. www.visionsofjoy.org

123. Smallwood, C. "The role of complementary and alternative medicine in the NHS: An investigation into the potential contribution of mainstream complementary therapies to healthcare in the UK." 2005. www.getwelluk.com/uploadedFiles/Publications/Smallwood

124. Jackson, E., P. McNeil, and L. Schlegel. "Does therapeutic touch help reduce pain and anxiety in patient's with cancer?" *Clinical Journal of Oncology Nursing* 12 (2008).

125. MORI Poll. *The Times*, 13 November 1989.

126. Thomas, K., and P. Coleman. "Use of complementary or alternative medicine in a general population in Great Britain: Results from the National Omnibus survey." Vol 26. no. 2. *Journal of Public Health* (Oxf), 2004.

127. Thomas, K. J., J. Carr, L. Westlake, and B. T. Williams. "Use of non-orthodox and conventional health care in Great Britain." *British Medical Journal* 302(6770) (1991).

128. Jackson, E. *Law and the Regulation of Medicines.* Bloomsbury, 2012.

129. www.bbc.co.uk/news/uk-england-birmingham-11434680

130. www.spiritualhealinganewfrontier.com

131. selbstgeheilt.com

132. Flatley, M. www.youtube.com/watch?v=McoSiK3T9hs (2013).

133. Ebdon, Peter. onedrive.live.com/?authkey=%21AAk4et%2DwJ2v6q%2DQ&cid=899C738DB4E3AF7C&id=899C738DB4E3A F7C%21124&parId= 899C738DB4E3AF7C%21121&o=OneUp. *Live Sport.* BBC. Radio 5, London. 16 May 2020.

134. Mentioned within Dr Craig Brown's presentation to the House of Lords.

135. Koenig, H. "Religion, Spirituality and Health; The Research and Clinical Implications."
International Scholarly Research Notices (2012).

136. J. Levin, *God, Faith & Health.* John Wiley & Sons (2002).

137. www.abraham-hicks.com

138. www.goodnewsnetwork.org

139. www.timwheater.com

140. www.hellinger.com

141. Jacobs, G. D. "Clinical applications of the relaxation response and mind–body interventions."
Journal of Alternative and Complementary Medicine 7 (2001); Lovallo, W. R. *Stress & Health;*
Biological and Psychological Interactions. Sage Publications, 2005.

142. Collins, F. S. *The Language of God: A Scientist Presents Evidence for Belief.* Pocket Books, 2007.

143. Landau, M. D. "Energy Healed Me — Over the Phone! A Scientist Explains How." *Huffington Post.*
19 October 2011. www.huffingtonpost.com/meryl-davids-landau/healing-over-the-phone_b_1011510.html

Recommended Reading

Bates, William. *Better Eyesight without Glasses.* Hyderabad: Orient Publishing, 2020.

Beckwith, Michael. *The Answer Is You.* Mumbai: Jaico, 2012.

Bloom, William. *The Endorphin Effect: A breakthrough strategy for holistic health and spiritual well-being.*
-London: Piatkus, 2001.

Braden, Gregg. *The Science of Self-Empowerment.* London: Hay House, 2017.

Braud, William. *Distant Mental Influence: Its Contributions to Science, Healing and Human Interactions.*
Charlottesville, VA: Hampton Roads Publishing, 2003.

Brinkley, Dannion. *Saved by the Light.* New York: HarperCollins, 1994.

Brofman, Martin. *Anything Can Be Healed.* Rochester, VT: Findhorn Press, 2019.

Byrne, Rhonda. *The Secret.* London: Simon & Schuster, 2006.

Chopra, Deepak. *Ageless Body, Timeless Mind.* London: Penguin, 2009.

Cousins, Norman. *Anatomy of an Illness: As Perceived by the Patient.*
New York: W.W. Norton & Co, 2005.

Diener, Ed, and Robert Biswas-Diener. *Happiness: Unlocking the Mysteries of Psychological Wealth.* Malden, MA: Blackwell Publishing, 2008.

Dossey, Larry. *One Mind: How Our Individual Mind Is Part of a Greater Consciousness and Why It Matters.* London: Hay House, 2013.

Dyer, Wayne W. *Wishes Fulfilled: Mastering the Art of Manifesting.* London: Hay House, 2012.

Eden, Donna, and David Feinstein. *Energy Medicine.* London: Piatkus Books, 1998.

Harvey, David. *The Power to Heal: An Investigation of Healing and the Healing Experience.* Wellingborough, UK: The Aquarian Press, 1983.

Hay, Louise. *You Can Heal Your Life.* Carlsbad, CA: Hay House, 1984.

Hicks, Esther, and Gerry Hicks. *The Law of Attraction.* Carlsbad, CA: Hay House, 2006.

Katie, Byron. *Loving What Is: Four Questions that Can Change Your Life.* London: Penguin, 2002.

Lawton, Ian. *The Power of You.* Rational Spirituality Press, 2014.

Linn, Denise. *How My Death Saved My Life.* Carlsbad, CA: Hay House, 2005.

Lipton, Bruce H. *The Biology of Belief.* London: Hay House, 2015.

Manning, Matthew. *The Healing Journey: A Step-by-Step Guide to Healing Yourself and Others.* London: Piatkus Books, 2001.

Moorjani, Anita. *Dying to Be Me.* London: Hay House, 2012.

Oschman, James. *Energy Medicine.* New York: Elsevier, 2016.

Sheldrake, Rupert. *Science and Spiritual Practices.* London: Hodder & Stoughton, 2017.

Siegel, Bernie. *The Art of Healing: Uncovering Your Inner Wisdom and Potential for Self Healing.* Navato, CA: New World Library, 2013.

Tolle, Eckhart. *The Power of Now.* London: Hodder & Stoughton, 2005.

Vitale, Joe, and Ihaleakala Hew Len. *Zero Limits: The Secret Hawaiian System for Wealth, Health, Peace, and More.* Hoboken, NJ: John Wiley & Sons, 2003.

Weil, Andrew. *Spontaneous Happiness.* London: Hodder & Stoughton, 2011.

Acknowledgements

One person cleared the way for me to be a volunteer healer at an NHS hospital. Better still, he allowed me to work in his clinic, which meant that he became personally aware of how healing affected his patients. He also agreed for me to conduct audits so that the healing effects that patients reported could be documented. When I alerted him to the opportunity of gaining research funding from the National Lottery, he brought together the necessary individuals and organizations to make a successful application. Dr Sukhdev Singh, a consultant physician at Good Hope Hospital and Senior Lecturer at the University of Birmingham Medical School, had the courage, drive and commitment to make all of this happen. Without his willingness to assess the value of healing for his patients, the research programme would not have happened, and this book could not have been written. I am indebted to Dr Singh for his kind and generous support, and for the joy it has brought me to work at his clinic. When I began writing, he gave me valuable advice, but he did not read the manuscript. I hope he approves of the book!

My sincere thanks go to all of the healers and individuals who have assisted in my endeavours to bring healing to the public. I would love to acknowledge everyone by name, but one person asked not to be mentioned. Consequently, I have referred only to those people whose involvement is already in the public domain. In particular, I thank David Daniels for his tremendous commitment to our voluntary healing group in Walsall. Despite a full-time profession and extended family commitments, he kept our dedicated team together for many years. He was also one of the main healers on the research trial.

For help with my two hospital audits, thanks go to Jan Lacy for producing the graphs, and to Marion Willberry for typing up hundreds of patient comments.

I was thrilled and touched when several long-time friends with professional skills in English volunteered to check my manuscript. Sian Davies read through the first draft, and could be objective, since she had no affinity to healing. But I then tinkered with the text and added more while waiting for the main research paper to be published. As explained in the book, the latter had to happen before I could go to print. Glynis Alder worked on the second draft – and in record time, because it seemed that the research paper was on the verge of being published. But more months passed, so I continued to add and amend. Then Patricia O'Grady read a proof copy and offered some beneficial ideas. Thank you, my friends.

I was a complete stranger to the two people I approached to read my first draft and write words of support – Dr Michael Dixon and the Duchess of Rutland. I felt honoured when they each readily emailed their agreement, and ecstatic when they provided glowing testimonials. Thank you, both. My gratitude also goes to the medical doctors, scientists and nurses who have chosen to buy a copy of my book and then sent me words of support for it.

My husband has never attempted to discourage me from being involved in healing or from embarking on healing-related projects. I am grateful for his continued support during the production of this book.

About the Author

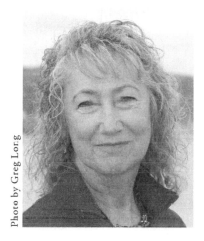

Photo by Greg Lorg

Sandy Edwards first trained to be a spiritual healer with The Healing Trust, a non-religious UK-based charity.

Now based in Dorset, she has been a volunteer healer for more than 20 years, seven of which were alongside a top consultant at a general hospital in Birmingham, UK. Her interest in promoting the benefits of healing and making it accessible to others led her to instigate the largest medical research trial of spiritual healing in the world.

To encourage others to seek healing, Sandy invites you to send your healing story to be included in her next book. You can remain anonymous, but if you are willing to be publicly identified, she will strive to team you up with a media contact so that others may learn of and be inspired by your story too.

https://www.facebook.com/healinginahospital
https://www.instagram.com/spiritualhealinginhospitals
Twitter : Sandy_E_Healing

For further information visit: **www.healinginahospital.uk**

Index

Also of Interest from Findhorn Press

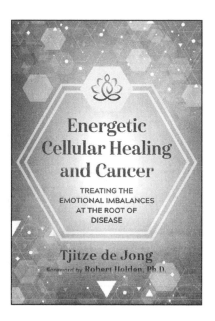

Energetic Cellular Healing and Cancer
Treating the Emotional Imbalances
at the Root of Disease
by Tjitze de Jong

OFFERING A GUIDE to the psychological causes of cancer and how energetic healing can assist in a mind-body cure, the author unravels the psychological aspects of an individual's energetic defense system and examines where possible energetic blocks might develop and how they can be dissolved.

978-1-64411-151-2

Also of Interest from Findhorn Press

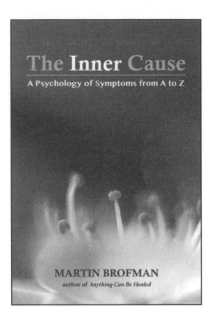

The Inner Cause
A Psychology of Symptoms from A to Z
by Martin Brofman

EXPLORING THE BODY as a map of consciousness, Martin Brofman explains how physical symptoms reflect stresses on your mind, emotions, and Spirit. In this book, he offers an A to Z compendium of 800 symptoms and a psychology of their inner causes, the messages they are trying to send to your consciousness.

978-1-84409-753-1

Also of Interest from Findhorn Press

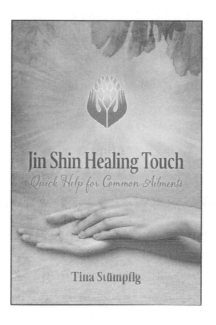

Jin Shin Healing Touch
Tina Stümpfig

JIN SHIN JYUTSU is an ancient Japanese healing art akin to an easier form of acupressure. This full color guide details the 52 energy points of Jin Shin Jyutsu and explains the sequence of points to hold to address specific ailments, conditions, and injuries and stimulate the body's self-healing response.

978-1-64411-076-8

FINDHORN PRESS

Life-Changing Books

Learn more about us and our books at
www.findhornpress.com

For information on the Findhorn Foundation:
www.findhorn.org